You and Neurosis

'*The grand aim of all science is to cover the greatest number of empirical facts by logical deduction from the smallest number of hypotheses or axioms.*'
                              ALBERT EINSTEIN

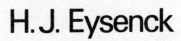

H. J. Eysenck

YOU AND NEUROSIS

Temple Smith
London

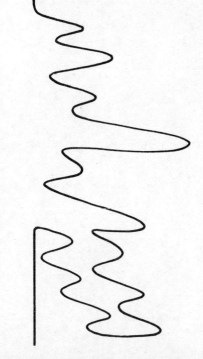

First published in Great Britain 1977
by Maurice Temple Smith Ltd
37 Great Russell Street, London WC1
© 1977 H. J. EYSENCK
ISBN 0 85117 1273
Typesetting by Input Typesetting Ltd
Printed in Great Britain by
Billing and Sons Ltd
Guildford, London and Worcester

Contents

Introduction   9

1 The Neurotic Paradox   15
  What is neurosis?   15
  Different types of neurosis   20
  How widespread is neurosis?   25
  Summary   35

2 Causes of Neurosis   37
  Demonology and psychoanalysis   37
  Biological factors   43
  Anxiety and conditioning   50

3 A Theory of Neurosis   61
  Watson's conditioning model   61
  A new model   72
  Personality and neurosis   89

4 Methods of Behaviour Therapy   107
  Desensitization   107
  Flooding   123
  Modelling   130

5 Asocial and Antisocial Behaviour   140
  The causes of criminality   140
  Aversion therapy   152
  Token economies   161

6 Neurosis and Society   170
  The effects of therapy   170
  The critics of behaviour therapy   187
  The ethics of behaviour therapy   196

Postscript: You and Neurosis   202

Bibliography   211

Index   217

Figures

1 The effects of different methods of treatment on nocturnal
  enuresis   46
2 Gradients of approach and avoidance   80
3 Reduction and enhancement of responses   85
4 Diathesis-stress model of neurosis   90
5 Modern model of personality, superimposed on the ancient
  'four temperaments' model   94
6 A hierarchical model of personality   96
7 The physiological basis of extraversion and neuroticism   103
8 Effects of 'flooding' type treatment   129
9 Reduction of time taken over compulsive rituals by patient
  after 'modelling' type treatment   133
10 Effects on frequency of headaches of three types of treatment   136
11 Improvement of seriously ill neurotic patients receiving no
   psychiatric treatment   172
12 Effects of behaviour therapy, psychotherapy and no treatment   182

Acknowledgements

The author acknowledges with thanks permission to quote material published by the following: Pergamon Press; American Psychological Association; Routledge & Kegan Paul; British Medical Journal.

To Sybil, who helped

Introduction

In this book I have tried to do something both difficult and presumptuous. As most readers will know, large numbers of people in the Western countries are falling prey to the various behavioural disorders that commonly come under the title of 'neurosis'; it is suggested by many psychiatrists that the numbers involved cover something like 30 per cent to 35 per cent of the total population. We shall presently look at the figures unearthed by research workers to see what truth there may be in this belief, and in the even more frequently voiced one that neurosis is a consequence of the stresses and strains of modern life, and is much more prevalent than it used to be. This latter proposition is very doubtful, but the prominence of neurosis among the disorders which lead people to consult their doctors is unquestioned.

Yet few people have any very clear idea of what precisely is meant by the term, neurosis; they do not know what causes neurotic disorders; and they have only very hazy views about the methods of treatment which are available. I have tried in this book to give an honest answer to these questions, in so far as such answers can at present be given, and I have also tried to indicate the sort of factual basis on which my answers are grounded. To those desperately worried and anxious about certain aspects of their lives I have tried to explain just what is causing their difficulties, and what they can do about them; the position of the neurotic has improved very greatly in recent years, and the hopes of a cure have advanced correspondingly.

Thus the major message of this book – if indeed it has a message, other than constituting a factual account – is a very positive one. We now understand, at least in principle, why people suffer from these mysterious disorders we call neuroses, and in the great majority of cases we can do something about them – not as a matter of several years of psychoanalysis, not as a matter of administering drugs such as tranquillizers, not as a matter of operating on the brain (leucotomy) or giving electric shocks to

9

the brain (ECT), but by simple behavioural re-education which, if it works at all, works in a relatively short period of time.

It is only honest to add at this point that what I have to say would not be accepted universally as being a correct and impartial statement of the truth. As is well known, there are many different schools advocating very different theories about the nature and origins of neurosis, and equally numerous groups offering equally different methods of treatment; *quot homines, tot sententiae!* Even if we only look at the psychoanalytic school, we find that it is splintered into innumerable sects and cliques, all at daggers drawn with each other. There are schools founded by rebels from the Freudian credo, like Jung and Adler; there are the neo-Freudians; there are followers of Stekel, of Reich, of Horney, of Sullivan, of Alexander, and of many other prophets. There are the 'physical' therapists, who pin their belief and hope on treatment by drugs, or by surgical interference.

How can the layman come to any reasonable conclusion about these many varied claims, without himself becoming an expert? The answer, to my mind, is very simple – oversimplified, critics will no doubt say. It is that by their fruits shall ye know them. Theories and methods which succeed in curing the neurotic of his or her complaints have something to teach us; theories and methods for which there is no evidence of success may not be completely wrong, but until they too can demonstrate beyond cavil their ability to succeed better than no treatment at all, or than simple medical, non-psychiatric treatment, they will be disregarded. This may seem a harsh doctrine, and desperately unfair to some otherwise very interesting speculations, but from the point of view of both science and the prospective patient it seems the only realistic way of dealing with what has become a major scandal. Theory-making there has to be in science, but theories have to retain some firm connection with hard fact. In the psychotherapeutic field this connection has become lost, and speculation is quite unfettered by demands for proof. This is an unhealthy situation, and the sooner it is ended, the better. We have come to the point where we are witnessing what T. H. Huxley used to call the tragedy of science: the slaying of a beautiful theory by an ugly fact. The beautiful theories are many; the ugly fact is that these theories do not work – they do not result in treatments which make the patient better.

There is another reason why I have become convinced that some theories are in fact better than others – apart from the fact that the treatments to which they give rise work, and can be seen to work. In science, application is preceded by extensive accumulation of knowledge in the laboratory; two thousand and more years of stellar observation, of laboratory experimentation, and of mathematical calculation preceded the application of all this knowledge to the conquest of interplanetary space, and the landing of man on the moon. Most psychiatric theories are *ad hoc* theories, not derived from systematic laboratory study, but introduced simply to explain the facts directly – either as they are, or as they are imagined to be. This is an unsafe and dangerous basis on which to proceed; there is certainly no precedent in physical science for such insouciance. If neurotic behaviour is acquired through some form of learning or conditioning (and it certainly is not due to physical lesions, which is the only rational alternative) then the knowledge accumulated over the past hundred years by psychologists of the laws concerning learning and conditioning should provide the main, or indeed the only, relevant body of knowledge from which to deduce theories concerning the origins and the treatment of neuroses. Modern learning theory is now in a position to provide such guidance, and this provenance of our knowledge makes it much less likely that our theories are mere speculation: they can be checked in the experimental laboratory, and amended or thrown out if they should prove erroneous. There is no such provision for the elimination of error in the case of the most popular psychiatric theories.

In what follows, I can, therefore, not promise to be unbiased, if by that we mean that all existing theories are discussed in an impartial manner. There are many books which attempt to do this; they invariably end up with a large number of undigested and indeed indigestible speculations, contradictory, without empirical support, and all unconnected with fundamental theory and experimentation. What I have tried to do has been quite different. I have tried to winnow the chaff from the grain; to retain what has both theoretical justification and practical support, but to jettison ruthlessly all else. In other words, I have presented what I consider at the moment the most likely and the most strongly supported view of what constitutes neurosis, what causes neurosis, and what may cure neurosis.

Such a view, at such a time, must inevitably be subjective to some extent; it is only fair to warn the reader of this subjectivity, and to add that many of the older and more experienced psychiatrists, psychoanalysts and psychotherapists would probably consider the views here put forward as unacceptable. Indeed, they mostly reject the criterion which I have suggested as being the most important one in judging between rival schools, namely actual success in treatment. To many psychiatrists, as we shall see, the 'symptoms' of which the patient complains are of little interest or importance; they are far more concerned with what they believe underlies these symptoms. This is an analogy from physical medicine; we do not treat the fever, and are not particularly interested in it. What we treat is the disease which produces the fever; cure that, and the fever itself vanishes. On this basis many psychotherapists disregard the 'symptoms' complained of by the patient, and concentrate on the elimination of the hypothetical 'complexes' supposed to lie at the basis of the neurosis. Unfortunately there is no acceptable, independent evidence of the existence of these 'complexes', and there is no evidence that their treatment through long-continued psychoanalysis, or shorter-term psychotherapy, actually has any influence on the 'symptoms'. This realization has considerably changed the claims made by psychiatrists for the alleged benefits of psychotherapy; it used to be claimed that these methods, and these methods alone, could cure patients suffering from neurotic disorders; nowadays it is claimed rather that their personalities are changed for the better in some mysterious way, and that they are better adapted to cope with the burden of their symptoms. Why they should be asked to do this when the symptoms can in fact be removed altogether by other methods is left unexplained.

It is difficult not to feel sympathy with neurotic patients, and indeed with the proverbial man in the street, who is mystified by the quarrels and disputations going on between 'experts' in the psychiatric field who seem unable to agree with each other. The present situation can only be understood once we realize that an old theory is dying and a new one is being born. As Max Planck, the great physicist and discoverer of the quantum theory, once said: 'A new scientific truth does not triumph by convincing its opponents and making them see the light, but rather because its opponents eventually die and a new generation grows up that is familiar with it.' If this is true in the 'hard' sciences, how much more is it true in the social sciences, which are notoriously 'soft' and resistant to experimentally ascertained fact. This book deals quite frankly with the new theory that is being born; the old is only mentioned in passing, to point contrasts and to deal with criticisms of the new made by the adherents of the old.

This may seem unfair discrimination, but in the same vein text-books of astronomy do not deal in detail with refutations of astrology, nor do textbooks of chemistry mention alchemists, except in passing. The bookstalls are full of popular accounts of psychoanalytic and other 'dynamic' writings; it would be a task of supererogation to duplicate what they have done so well. Readers who wish to learn about these older theories will have no difficulty at all in becoming acquainted with them, in all their different varieties. It is because there is no book outlining the new theories that I have written this one, making a quite conscious choice in delimiting the discussion and excluding detailed refutations and appraisals of older theories. My purpose was not an overall appraisal of what psychiatrists of one kind or another believe and do, but simply an exposition of what I believe has now been shown to be the most reasonable, adequate and promising theory of neurosis in existence.

That does not mean that it is perfect, or that it cannot be improved, or even that it will not be replaced in due course by another theory altogether. Theories are inventions of the human mind, never adequate to cover the multiplicity of events occurring in nature; as long as they account for the invariant properties of naturally occurring phenomena in a given field, and make predictions which, when tested experimentally or clinically, are borne out, so long are they useful and acceptable. Once they fall, they have to be replaced. Freudianism has failed; there can be no question of that. As Sir Peter Medawar, Nobel Laureate in Medicine, once put it: 'Considered in its entirety, psychoanalysis won't do. It is an end-product, moreover, like a dinosaur or a zeppelin; no better theory can ever be erected on its ruins, which will remain for ever one of the saddest and strangest of all landmarks in the history of twentieth-century thought.' This premature crystallization of spurious orthodoxies has cast its mythological spell over psychiatry for too long; the time has come for innovative treatments and new thinking.

How did it ever happen that notoriously poor theories (judged by the ordinary standards of the philosophy of science), giving rise to equally notoriously unsuccessful methods of treatment, ever cast this spell, and were accepted by presumably hard-headed physicians? The great Louis Pasteur, who almost single-handedly created modern medicine, had the answer: 'Physicians are inclined to engage in hasty generalizations. Possessing a natural or acquired distinction, endowed with a quick intelligence, an elegant and facile conversation, the more eminent they are, the less leisure do they have for investigative work. Eager for knowledge, they are apt too readily to accept attractive but inadequately proven theories.' Alas, physicians were not alone in this; many literary and artistic people followed suit, seduced by the high literary qualities of Freud's and, to a lesser extent, Jung's writings. With these we cannot compete; we shall have to rest our case on the facts presented in this book.

1 The Neurotic Paradox

What is neurosis?

Considering the very frequent use of the term 'neurosis' by psychiatrists and laymen alike, one might expect that its meaning was clear-cut, and that a definition could easily be produced. This is not so; indeed, it is doubtful if there really is such a 'thing' as neurosis at all, and if there is, it will prove quite difficult to tie it down. 'Neurosis' is of course a concept, and concepts have no real existence – in the sense that tables and chairs, pigs and cows, walruses and carpenters can be said to exist. (Even with these fairly substantial objects and bodies, professional philosophers raise difficulties about 'existence', but for our purpose we may disregard these.) Intelligence is a concept, so is gravitation, or heat, or electricity; such concepts summarize individual experiences sharing something in common. The concept 'intelligence' summarizes individual occasions of successful or unsuccessful problem-solving; 'gravitation' individual occasions of bodies falling, or otherwise attracting each other; 'heat' individual occasions where two bodies exchange molecular motion, and so on. 'Neurosis' is a term we often use for behaviour which is associated with strong emotion, which is maladaptive, and which the person giving rise to it realizes is nonsensical, absurd, or irrelevant, but which he is powerless to change. Phobic fears of darkness, cats, heights, open spaces, enclosed spaces or any number of stimuli which are not only harmless, but which are realized to be truly so by the person experiencing that fear may serve as an example. Another is obsessive-compulsive behaviour, in which fear of dirt and contamination leads to ever-repeated handwashing and other ceremonial behaviour, so much so that the sufferer can hardly do anything else all day and is completely incapacitated. Strong depressive reactions to events where the emotion is incommensurate with the seriousness of the event provoking it is a third. We shall discuss the different varieties of neurosis later on, as well as the characteristics which

15

tie them together; here let us merely note the ever-present elements of emotion, maladaptiveness, and relative insight shown by the patient.

This element of insight is extremely important; the neurotic typically knows that his behaviour is irrational, counter productive, and against his own best interests. He does it because he cannot help himself. He has insight into his condition in the sense that he knows perfectly well that something is wrong; he simply cannot do anything to help himself. He feels himself dragged along by a flood of emotional impulses which he is powerless to control, and he cries out for help in this agonizing situation. Few things are more terrifying than being subject to damaging forces which we cannot understand or control; that is precisely the position of the neurotic, and in this he clearly differs from the non-neurotic or 'normal' person. Actually we shall see that the distinction is not absolute. We all behave occasionally in less than rational ways; we all are controlled to some extent by our emotions; we often behave in ways that are less than optimally adaptive – and we often realize that this is so and deplore our own 'stupidity'. (The term is put in inverted commas because it signifies something other than the opposite of 'intelligence' – highly intelligent people are not protected from emotional troubles in the slightest degree, and neurosis strikes among the bright and the dull alike. We sometimes call ourselves 'stupid' because we know that we could and should have done better, not because we lacked the necessary IQ!) Thus there may be a continuum, ranging from the most stable to the most unstable or neurotic; there may not be an absolute point at which we may say that those to the left are 'normal' and those to the right 'neurotic'. The difficulty is precisely the same as that we would encounter if we were asked to make an absolute distinction between people who were tall and people who were short; the difference is real but any absolute cutting point is arbitrary.

It is very important to realize that there is a very definite distinction between neurosis and another psychiatric type of abnormality which is commonly referred to as psychosis. There are several different types of functional psychoses – a term indicating that these mental disorders are not produced by detectable lesions in the nervous system, or by other physical factors, but are 'functional' in the sense that they can only be detected by the aberrant functioning of the patient in the social world. Psychoses are much more serious than most neuroses, and fortunately they are much rarer; only something like two or three per cent of the population is likely to suffer from attacks of schizophrenia or manic-depressive psychosis, the two most frequent functional psychoses.

Psychoses, although they are called 'functional', are almost certainly based on inherited chemical malfunctioning of the metabolic system; these chemical errors provide the background which is needed for various social stresses to produce the final, tragic end result. No such chemical errors are likely to be present in the neurotic, and the causation of his troubles is quite different. Psychotics typically have little or no insight. The schizophrenic who proclaims that he is Napoleon or that he is in mental telepathic communication with the President of the United States; the psychotic depressive who believes that his insides are rotting, or that he is responsible for all the evil in the world, are 'mad' in the common meaning of the term. They lack insight into their condition, and indeed this lack of insight is a major part of their illness.

The evidence which shows that neurosis and psychosis are very different disorders is very strong; yet there are still many psychiatrists, particularly psychoanalysts, who deny this. According to Freud, all mental disorder is a regression to infantile modes of adjustment; the further the regression proceeds, the more serious the disorder. Neurosis is characteristic of a lesser retreat, psychosis of a major one; there is no real distinction between the two, other than degree of regression. This is an appealing idea, simplifying matters were it but true; unfortunately the evidence is entirely the other way. I shall just sketch briefly the reasons why this notion is unacceptable.

(1) First is the genetic evidence. Among the close and not-so-close relatives of psychotics there are found many other psychotics (not necessarily showing the same type of psychosis); there are also found many abnormal people who are schizoid (i.e. whose behaviour resembles that of schizophrenics, without being so seriously disordered that they can be classified as psychotic), psychopathic and criminal, alcoholic, etc. What is lacking, and what should be there if Freud were right, is a surplus of neurotics; these are conspicuously missing. Conversely, among

the close relatives of known neurotics we find many other neurotics, but no surplus of psychotics. Thus there are two great 'Erbkreise' (genetic circles – the German word is often used because it was largely German psychiatrists and geneticists who clarified these points in the 1920s and afterwards). There is a psychotic one and a neurotic one, both being independent of the other.

(2) Second comes the evidence from biochemical and neurophysiological investigations of psychotics, and the comparison of the findings from these patients with findings on neurotics and normals. This is not the place to go into details, but it has been found that there are various peculiarities and abnormalities in the blood serum, the sweat and the urine of psychotics (particularly schizophrenics) which are not found in neurotics or normals. There is no neurophysiological or biochemical sign that *absolutely* distinguishes psychotics and neurotics, or psychotics and normals; psychiatrists are working on this, and we shall have to await the success of their labours. But we already know pretty well that neurotics have nothing in common with psychotics along these lines.

(3) The third difference emerges from studies of neural reactivity, that is, the reactions of the nervous system when stressed. This can be measured along many different lines. We may measure the changes in pupil size in the dark-adapted eye when the subject is stressed through sudden immersion of his arm in ice-cold water. We may measure the flurry of brain-waves that are recorded on the electroencephalograph when a sudden sound breaks the quiet of the laboratory (the so-called evoked potentials). Or we can study the 'sedation threshold', the response of the organism to intravenous injections of drugs such as sodium amytal. Along all these lines, there are profound differences between psychotic and neurotic patients, with the neurotic behaving very much like the normal person, and the psychotic being the odd man out.

(4) Even on rather bizarre measures psychotics behave differently from neurotics. It is well established that psychotics (including others in their 'Erbkreise', such as psychopaths) tend to be born more frequently than other groups during the first few months of the year; this is not true of neurotics, who show no difference from normals.

(5) There are, in addition to these biological differences, many clinical ones. On Freud's theory, psychotics should pass through a neurotic phase before falling ill, and they should behave neurotically when recovering from their psychosis. This is not usually so. A psychotic does not normally behave neurotically prior to, or subsequent to, his illness. Neurotics do not usually develop into psychotics. There are individual cases which seem to contradict this rule; in some people we seem to detect the presence of both psychosis and neurosis. There is no reason why this should not be so; a person may have both malaria and a broken toe. This does not prove that a broken toe is an early phase of malaria.

(6) Day-to-day variations in the behaviour of neurotics are usually related to antecedent changes in environmental conditions; this is hardly ever so in the behaviour of psychotics. For them, the controlling factors are seemingly internal, in a way characteristic of organically determined conditions. Hence even when we are dealing with the same apparent symptom, for example depression, there are clear-cut differences. These are reflected in the nomenclature used. Neurotic depression is called 'reactive depression' (because it represents a reaction to external events, though it may be an exaggerated reaction); psychotic depression is called 'endogenous depression', because it is internal and not responsive to changes in outside conditions.

(7) The effects of psychological treatment, whether psychotherapy or behaviour therapy, are very different in the two sets of conditions. Psychotics hardly respond at all, as would be expected from what was said above in point (6); neurotics seem much more reactive, and do often recover (although, as we shall see, the degree to which this recovery is due to the treatment is still a moot point).

(8) Psychological tests, representing a great variety of verbal and behavioural situations and responses, have been applied in great profusion to psychotics and neurotics. The outcome has been very clear-cut. Tests which differentiate normals from psychotics do not differentiate normals from neurotics, and tests which differentiate neurotics from normals do not differentiate psychotics from normals. In other words, neurotics and psychotics both differ from normals, but they do so along quite different dimensions of constitution, of reaction and of

behaviour. These eight differences are not the only ones which
could be listed, but they will suffice to indicate that the view of a
single continuum from normal, through neurotic, to psychotic, is
no longer tenable. We shall be dealing in this book almost entirely with neurotic disorders; psychology does not, at the moment,
make any clear contribution to the treatment of psychotics. Its
relevance is largely to the treatment of neurotics.

Different types of neurosis

One of the difficulties attending the notion of 'neurosis' is the
fact that what are called neurotic disorders present a very
variegated field of seemingly unrelated symptoms. Psychiatrists
often speak of various syndromes, such as anxiety state, reactive
depression, fatigue syndrome, hypochondria, hysteria, psychasthenia, obsessional-compulsive personality, and many more.
When encountered in the textbooks these can be described and
no doubt present a reasonably orderly picture, but in actual fact
few patients fall clearly and cleanly into one or the other of these
categories; most show symptoms characteristic of more than one
syndrome and some show symptoms from all. Even worse: a person who at one time may seem to fall fairly clearly into one
group may at another time fall into quite a different one.

This has led to a great and widely recognized weakness of psychiatric diagnostic methods: different psychiatrists, diagnosing
the same set of patients, come up with quite divergent diagnostic
labels for the same people. Many experiments have been carried
out in an effort to make this more precise as a statement, and the
outcome has always been the same. When well-trained psychiatrists, who have received the same sort of training and have
agreed on definitions of the various categories, are asked to give
diagnoses of one and the same set of patients, independently of
each other, agreement is seldom better than 20 per cent – leaving
80 per cent to chance, to individual biases and notions, and other
irrelevant factors. Agreement on whether a particular illness is
neurotic as opposed to psychotic is of course better than that, but
even here there are many sources of disagreement, some of them
quite far-reaching. Thus American psychiatrists have a very extended concept of schizophrenia, embracing many other psychotic and neurotic states that in Britain and Europe generally
would be diagnosed as depressive, or psychopathic, or hysterical.

In one study, comparing diagnostic habits in the USA and in Britain, similar groups of patients (and in one case an identical group of patients) were diagnosed as schizophrenic five times as frequently by the psychiatrists trained in the USA as by those trained in Britain! Thus the nationality of the psychiatrists was far more important than the disease of the patient in deciding the diagnosis. This must give one pause in taking diagnoses too seriously.

At first sight such general notions as the absence of insight in psychotics might seem to furnish one with an adequate, and indeed infallible, criterion; second thoughts suggest that this is far from the case. A paranoid patient complains that he is being persecuted by his employers, or by the police. He may be making all this up, in which case he could be genuinely diagnosed as paranoid. But he may also be telling the truth; some people have in the past been persecuted by employers and police, for one reason or another. How can we decide, without a major detective enquiry into all the circumstances of the case? Even worse, it may be true that the patient in question is being persecuted, but he may have brought this persecution upon himself by his paranoid behaviour in the first place. Given that the psychiatrist has only a very limited amount of time to spend on each patient, and that social workers also cannot expend unlimited resources on investigating the complex and seemingly endless ramifications of each case, it will be obvious that our criterion of 'insight' may in actual fact be quite difficult to apply. Of course in most cases the truth is pretty obvious, but it is the not-so-obvious cases which cause embarrassing difficulties in diagnosis – and unfortunately it is these that constitute such a large proportion of the psychiatrist's work.

Having noted these weaknesses in psychiatric diagnosis – weaknesses which do not diminish the need for a good diagnostic system, of course, but which point to the need for a drastic revision of existing ones – we may say that neurotic illnesses seem to fall into two major groups. The existence of these groups was originally suggested by the great French psychiatrist Pierre Janet, and later on linked by C. G. Jung with the major personality types of extraversion and introversion. Extraverts, Jung suggested, tended to have hysterical personality types and develop hysterical conversion symptoms when neurotic. This means that they tend to be histrionic, outgoing, with quick mood changes, exaggerated emotional reactions. Neurotic symptoms will tend to be of a psychosomatic kind, i.e. they will tend to mimic bodily disfunctions. Glove or stocking anaethesia are typical of these; the patient will have no feeling in the hand or the leg over roughly the area occupied by glove or stocking, but not coinciding at all with the areas known to be served by sets of ascending neurones. Many other bodily disfunctions can be so imitated, from headaches to cardiac disorders; indeed, it is often difficult to know whether a symptom is hysterical or genuine. The term 'conversion symptoms' is sometimes used to indicate that the patient has converted a mental disability into a physical one, making him curiously detached and non-anxious in his behaviour. The term 'belle indifference' was coined to characterize this lack of (appropriate) anxiety. Also in this ex-traverted group we have psychopaths, people lacking in social responsibility, without conscience, and without guilt feelings; these often become criminals. Psychosomatic disorders proper, about which we shall be hearing more later on, also often come into this group. What is characteristic of these various syndromes is the fact that these patients are 'acting out'; they turn their dis-order outwards, towards other people. Their symptoms are out-wardly apparent and indeed obvious; they tend to blame the out-er world, rather than themselves, and they trick and punish other people for their own misfortune.

Introverts, Jung suggested, tended to be psychasthenics; this term is now obsolete, and has been replaced by such words as anxiety state and dysthymia. Essentially, it denotes a state of weakness due to emotional excess; a psychasthenic is a person so overcome by anxiety, fear, phobic reactions and other emotional excesses that he is not fit to pursue a normal course of existence. These anxieties and fears may be localized, and indeed there are such things as monosymptomatic phobias – a person may be terribly afraid of snakes, or cats, or heights, so much so that his whole life is governed by this fear. More usually, there are many diverse fears; these may be of people, of situations or of certain classes of objects. Sometimes they may be quite diffuse and difficult to recognize; fear of the future, of annihilation, of death, or even of existence as such may be observed. Many of these situations or objects cause fear in ordinary people who are not neurotics; the difference lies in the *strength* of these neurotic fears, their *persistence,* and the inability of the patient to act normally in spite of them. Many people are worried about the atomic bomb, but they do not go to the extreme of changing their whole course of living on that basis. It is these exaggerated emotions and reactions which are so characteristic of the neurotic, particularly the introverted, 'psychasthenic' neurotic.

Obsessive-compulsive patients also have strong, in fact over-strong emotional reactions, but they tend to perform certain actions which almost in a magical fashion serve as a defence against these fears. Thus a person may be terribly afraid of dirt and contamination; whenever he is in a situation in which he may come into contact with dirt, excreta, or even dust and such unavoidable objects as other people, his fear of contamination can only be allayed if he can go and thoroughly wash himself; he may take a very long time over this, and the very next occasion where he encounters possible contamination leads to another bout of washing, cleansing, drying and so on. This behaviour reduces his anxiety, but of course it fatally disrupts his life; he can no longer work, indulge in any sort of sport or other pastime, and even his love-life is incredibly complicated. Some obsessive-compulsive patients are ruminators; they constantly go back over their ideas, in case they might have made a mistake in coming to conclusions. Many go back over their past actions; they check dozens of times whether they have locked the doors at night; they go over additions and other calculations time and time again to make quite sure they are right, and so on. A mild degree of such obsessive-compulsive behaviour may be quite useful in accountants, bank clerks and other people whose job requires unusual accuracy, but as shown by patients this is clearly a grave personality disorder. If only, one often feels, one could take an average of the careless, impulsive, extraverted hysteric and the overcareful, obsessional, introverted compulsive patient!

These, of course, are extremes; many neurotic patients, perhaps the majority, are in between the typically extraverted and the typically introverted groups, and show a variety of symptoms which are pretty specific to their circumstances, without giving rise to descriptive epithets like 'hysterical' or 'obsessive-compulsive'. It is these who make diagnosis so difficult; if our clinical population only consisted of hysterics and obsessive-compulsives, how easy life would be. Even so, diagnosis within the field of neurosis is probably not very important. Most neurotics obviously have something wrong with them; indeed, they usually come flocking to the doctor, or the psychiatric hospital, to complain of whatever it is, and once psychosis of any kind is excluded the treatment which is appropriate is decided much more by the specific symptom shown, and the circumstances of their lives, than by any diagnosis, however correct.

We are not as yet concerned with the problem of treatment, however; we are still in the middle of a discussion of the nature of the neurotic paradox. Why is it that neurosis has puzzled so many doctors and scientists for such a long time; why is it that people show a fear and a dislike of neurosis which is hardly justified in comparison with other, more terrible diseases; why is it that the very mention of mental disorder causes an uneasy silence to fall over most groups in whose discussion the concept happens to come up? The answer probably is that we fear most what we do not understand and cannot control; knowledge enables us to understand, to look ahead, and to plan counteractions. Where we seem helpless, rational reactions are useless, superstition takes over, and ancient fears recur. Neurosis seems unintelligible, threatening, and alien to our nature because it clearly contains a paradox. Our normal existence is governed by some form of hedonic calculus, as is that of any animal. We persist in those activities which in the past have resulted in reward, or positive reinforcement, as the psychologist often terms it; we desist from activities which in the past have resulted in punishment, or negative reinforcement. What constitutes reward and punishment for any particular person may differ profoundly; the martyr may prefer the crown of thorns, the epicure the twelve-course meal. But each person knows (or thinks he knows) just what it is that would satisfy him; and, given the choice, he knows what he wants and grabs it. There are of course frequent conflicts, as when choosing A means giving up B, or when choosing A means having to submit to C; nevertheless, where a person has a choice, he tends to choose that which he prefers. He may of course be wrong, and regret bitterly afterwards having made one choice rather than another; nevertheless, at the time of making the choice he did what he wanted — or at least what he thought he wanted.

This is not true of the neurotic. In his case, he wants A, but does B. He wants to get on in life, work hard and get somewhere in his job; he certainly does not want to spend his life washing his hands and be out of a job with his home crumbling around him. He wants to lead a normal life, not sit at home all day because of some silly fear of cats which makes it impossible to go out in case he might meet one – particularly when he knows full well that cats are really not dangerous at all. He (or more frequently she) is leading a life which he or she would never have chosen, and the more negative the reinforcement, the greater is the strength with which he or she embraces this particular kind of life. In other words, the neurotic chooses to do A but does B; the more he does B, which he dislikes and finds punishing, the more does he go on doing it! The greater his desire to do A, the less seems to be his ability to carry out his wishes. He acts in exact contrariety to his wishes and desires; yet he goes on doing so, year after year. He undergoes terrible suffering, yet this suffering does not bring him any gains. This is the neurotic paradox, and for the sufferer it is a very damaging and cruel hoax indeed. We shall see in the next chapter what theories have been proposed to explain the mystery; in this section we shall merely rest content with the exposition of its nature.

How widespread is neurosis?

There is a widespread belief that neuroses are far more common now than they used to be; this is usually attributed to the 'stresses and strains' which are supposed to characterize modern life. On *a priori* grounds, this sounds a very unlikely story. Compared to people living even one or two hundred years ago, we are remarkably mollicoddled, protected, and kept from any real 'stresses and strains'. Medicine was in its infancy a hundred years ago, with anaesthetics hardly in use; indeed, physicians probably did more harm than good. Dentistry was a bad joke, consisting of little more than extractions performed at fair grounds, with the victim anaesthetised by gin. Infant mortality was tragically high, and the average length of life was much below our present three-score years and ten. Poverty was widespread and cruel, to an extent that we can hardly even imagine. The class system was much firmer, and rebellion impossible. Sex roles were immutable, or nearly so, with much consequent suffering.

Transport was only for the rich, and even for them it was inconvenient, slow and uncomfortable. The feudal society repressed and disdained the vast majority of the Queen's subjects, while calling upon them for supreme sacrifices during inhumanly cruel wars.

And this was a golden age in comparison to even earlier times – the times of Attila the Hun, of the Black Death, of invasions and war, followed by plunder, rape and slavery. In those years famine stalked the land, either following the war-like hordes of invaders, or arriving unsolicited in the footsteps of natural disasters. These were real stresses and strains, in comparison with which our modern complaints seem childish and totally uncalled for. Modern life is as free from adversity as life has ever been, and particularly in the Western world the welfare state has encompassed us all in a web of paternalism which if anything threatens to kill our independence and ability to fashion our own defences against adversity.

But these are just arguments; what are the facts? These are remarkably difficult to come by, for obvious reasons. The recognition of the various types of neurosis is a fairly recent achievement; it is difficult to recognize our neurosis in the descriptions of ancient ills. Even where this is possible, there is little quantitative information to be had of days gone by. Such information as we have deals almost exclusively with middle or upper-class people; the vast majority led lives unchronicled and unsung – and largely unobserved by physicians. Coming to our own days, it is still remarkably difficult to find agreement even on simple questions, such as the number of neurotics in a given country or district. The reason for this is of course quite plain. Neurotic disorders, as we have seen, range along a dimension from (almost perfect) normality, through mild and not-so-mild to severe and extremely severe forms; there is no point where we can say that on the one side are neuroses, on the other normality. Just as we cannot say what proportion of the population is tall, the borderline being arbitrary between tall and short, so we cannot say what proportion is neurotic; we can take an arbitrary cut and try to define this as closely as may be, but our figures will never be able to pretend to any great accuracy. However, in broad outline it is possible to get some sort of overview of the situation, and this is what is being attempted in this section.

Let us start with a look into history – going as far back as seems reasonable. The book which I shall quote is entitled *The English malady: Or a treatise of nervous disease of all kinds, as spleen, vapours, lowness of spirits, hypochondrial and hysterical distempers, etc.* It was written by G. Cheyne in 1733, about 250 years ago, and published in London by Strahand and Leake. This is what the author had to say:

> The Moisture of our Air, the Variableness of our Weather (from our situation amidst the Ocean) the Rankness and Fertility of our Soil, the Richness and Heaviness of our Food, and Wealth and Abundance of the Inhabitants (from their universal Trade) the Inactivity and sedentary Occupations of the better Sort (among whom this Evil mostly rages) and the Humour of living in great, populous and consequently unhealthy Towns, have brought forth a Class and Set of Distempers, with atrocious and frightful Symptoms, scarce known to our Ancestors, and never rising to such fatal Heights, nor afflicting such Numbers in any other known Nations. These nervous Disorders being computed to make almost one third of the Complaints of the People of Condition in England.

Thus in the golden age of England one person in three (of the better sort, at least) was suffering from recognizable neurotic disorders, diagnosed under the rather unfamiliar headings of spleen, vapours, etc. This figure is remarkably similar to the most modern figures relating to our own times.

Not only is the estimate of prevalence similar to that given recently by a working party of College of General Practitioners; the very notions about the causation of mental illness mentioned have persisted to this day. There is the belief that mental disorders are increasing as a result of our decadent, sedentary, unhealthy mode of life; that they are associated with dampness, the climate and overcrowding; that they are more common here than elsewhere, and that they are more common than they once were. There is no evidence for any of these beliefs, then as now; these are not the causal factors which we shall find responsible for neurotic disorders when we turn to a proper discussion of this topic.

But all this is history; what about the prevalence of neurosis in our time? There are several good studies here, and if they seem to give widely different answers, there are reasons for this which suggest that disagreement is perhaps less than it appears to be at first sight. Let us begin with a look at neurosis in mental hospitals. These are devoted largely to the most serious types of mental illness, mainly psychotic ones; neurotics are usually admitted to outpatient treatment, and make up something like a quarter of all diagnoses. However, many anxiety neuroses are camouflaged by physical symptoms, and may be seen in other departments; thus among patients with cardiovascular symptoms seen in a cardiology practice, anxiety states were diagnosed in 10 to 14 per cent of all cases. These figures do not give at all a fair representation of the amount of neurotic illness; many quite severely ill neurotics shy away from going to 'loony bins' for diagnosis and treatment, knowing full well that they are not 'mad' (in the sense of being psychotic). Hence they often suffer in silence, ignorant of other alternatives and reluctant to see a doctor at all.

During the war, it became clear that neurotic illnesses were responsible for a considerable amount of absence from work, and a special study was done of some 3,000 workers in light and medium engineering factories. During the six month period of the study, 9 per cent of the men and 13 per cent of the women were found to have suffered from definite and disabling neurotic illness (anxiety states, mild depressive states, obsessional states and hysteria). A further 19 per cent of men and 23 per cent of women had experienced episodes of minor neurosis. Neurotic illness caused something like 30 per cent of all absence from work due to illness and represented an annual loss of 3 working days for men and 6 for women. Wartime factors, such as bombing etc., were not particularly prominent, and although hours were long, wages were high, and redundancy was not a problem. Altogether some 28 per cent of men, and some 36 per cent of women, were plagued by neurotic symptoms strong enough to be recognised by the interviewing doctor; this sex difference emerges again and again, with women always the more 'neurotic' sex. Cheyne's estimate of one in three does seem to apply, even though these men and women were not of the 'better sort'.

This study was done in England; a much more thorough and

detailed study in Norway, also carried out during the war, but in a remote rural district, gave similar results. A quarter of the population showed gross psychological abnormality at some time during the five years of observation. This estimate was based on detailed psychiatric interviews carried out by an experienced psychiatrist.

Peacetime studies have largely concentrated on patients consulting their GP, in an effort to estimate the incidence of neurosis in general practice. One large-scale study concluded that about one fifth of patients seen in any one day in an urban practice were suffering from stress disorders. Such figures depend very much on what is included in the definition. Thus in another study, it was found that prevalence rates of about 5 per cent were found if strict criteria as laid down in the International Classification of Diseases were used. This rate rose to 9 per cent when criteria were loosened to include all patients who showed 'conspicuous psychiatric morbidity', by which was meant overt psychological disturbance regardless of diagnosis. Including patients with physical symptoms for which no organic cause was detectable raised the incidence to 38 per cent, and including all patients with psychosomatic disorders, such as peptic ulcer and asthma, brought it to a staggering total of 52 per cent, suggesting that over half of all the disorders seen by the GP were either psychiatric, or had a strong psychiatric component. These figures illustrate the difficulty of obtaining any very accurate estimate of the incidence of such a protean thing as neurosis.

A similar study, using general practitioners in London and sampling every eighth patient's case notes from the practitioners' medical records, was carried out by M. Shepherd and his colleagues at the Maudsley Hospital. They tried to estimate the prevalence rate over one year for adults who sought help for psychiatric problems, and found that psychiatric morbidity was one of the commonest reasons for consultation, particularly among women. Psychosis accounted for something like $\frac{1}{2}$ per cent of the consultations; neurosis for 9 per cent (6 per cent for men, 12 per cent for women). Conditions associated with psychiatric disorder accounted for another 5 per cent. Thus among patients consulting their doctor, the incidence of neurosis is apparently much less than the 30 per cent or so we have encountered in general surveys; the reason presumably must be that many people who are suffering from neurotic and other psychiatric disorders do not consult their doctor, but suffer in silence. It is interesting that it has been found that differences in attitude among practitioners are very important in determining differences observed in prevalence rates; GPs sympathetic to emotional problems tend to have much higher prevalence rates than GPs not so sympathetic.

Prevalence rates at any moment of time do not tell us the probability that a given person might at some stage of his life have a nervous breakdown or other form of psychiatric illness. A large-scale study in Sweden, undertaken by Essen-Möller and later continued by Hagnell, gave some startling answers to this question. Lifetime prevalence of psychosis was found to be 1.7 per cent, and for neurosis 13.1 per cent. The risk of developing mental illness over a ten-year period (mainly neurotic, of course) was 11.3 per cent for men and 20.4 per cent for women. The estimated cumulative lifetime risk up to the age of 60 years was 43.4 per cent for the men, and a staggering 73.0 per cent for the women! These figures include mild forms of neurosis; when we only include mental illnesses associated with severe impairment of function the figures are 7.9 per cent for men and 15.4 per cent for women. These are indeed frightening figures, and they indicate that mental illness is almost omnipresent, if only in its milder forms; half the members of the population are subject to an attack at some time or other of their lives.

Several total prevalence studies have been carried out in the United States; the universal result has been that the wider the criteria, and the more intensive the methods used for ascertaining cases, the larger the proportion of the population regarded as subject to mental disorder. In one such study in Stirling County, 58 per cent were regarded as 'genuine psychiatric cases'. In a study in Midtown Manhattan, 23 per cent of the population were suggested to be suffering from serious psychiatric symptoms and some degree of impaired functioning. When more conservative criteria are used, figures vary from 6 per cent in Baltimore, through 9 per cent in the same town, to 14 per cent in New Jersey. American results, both in the absolute figures and in their variability, agree well with those reported from England and Scandinavia.

These varied figures may leave a confused impression; they vary so much because of different standards of diagnosis, different criteria employed, different locations, and different time-periods spanned. It is worth describing in some detail a particular study which may bring home to readers the precise nature of the problem. The study was done by Taylor and Chave in England; it involved recording the prevalence of mental illness in the community at large, in general practice, and in hospital practice. Three separate areas were chosen, in the expectation that different rates would be found. One was a satellite New Town (called 'Newton'), which was a socially planned community with full local working opportunities. The second was a dormitory housing estate ('Outlands'), which had good living accommodation but poor social facilities and no local work. The third ('Oldfield') was a decaying area of London, with poor housing and a slum mentality. The major question asked was whether a 'good community' promoted mental health and well being, or whether genetic and constitutional factors were more important. Table 1 gives the answers found in random sample interviews carried out in these three places. It will be seen that nervous symptoms are reported by about one in three of the adults interviewed, and that this figure is about the same for all three samples. Again Cheyne is vindicated, apparently. The figures were about twice as high for females as for males, and they seem to indicate that long-standing or constitutional factors are of much greater importance in producing neurotic symptoms than are environmental ones. This conclusion is of course only very

Table 1

Symptoms	Percentage of Adults reporting:		
	Newton	Outlands	Oldfield
'Nerves'	18%	22%	24%
'Depression'	17%	17%	12%
'Sleeplessness'	10%	12%	10%
'Undue irritability'	13%	11%	8%
At least one of these:	33%	35%	31%

tentative; we shall return to the role of heredity in a later chapter. The environmental factors here studied may of course not have been the important ones, although they were those that have often been singled out as responsible for at least certain types of neurotic illness.

During any one year, about 8 per cent of the inhabitants of Newton were treated for neurosis; this took the form mainly of anxiety and tension states. Such a figure of course implies a much higher figure for longer periods – say ten years, or even a lifetime; it is compatible with the Swedish estimates already quoted. This minor disease was not found to be related to length of residence or income. It represented, Taylor and Chave concluded, 'a deeply embedded pattern within the nervous system'; the step from subclinical syndrome to overt neurosis occurred when the patient took note of the subjective symptoms and consulted a doctor. This overt neurotic group, they state, varies in size according to the quantity and quality of general practice and specialist psychiatric services available. This view agrees well with an almost universal finding, namely a sort of Parkinson's Law of neurosis – the more psychiatric services are provided, the more mental illness will come to the fore. Put in another way, *the number of people seeking help for their neurotic problems in any population expands to take up all psychiatric care that is available.*

One final study may be worth mentioning, as this used a properly validated anxiety questionnaire (the Morbid Anxiety Inventory or MAI), and was carried out on a proper random sample of the British population by the Gallup Poll Organization. On this questionnaire, scores above 17 are fairly sure indices of clinical anxiety, with scores between 14 and 17 constituting an in-between ground between anxiety and fair degree of normality. Twenty-nine per cent of the subjects questioned had been treated for 'worry, depression or any other nervous complaint'; again we find this magic figure of one in three. Taking the score of 14 and above as evidence of anxiety, 44 per cent of the sample turned out to be anxious; if we use the more conservative score of 17, the figure falls to 31 per cent, similar to Taylor and Chave's estimate for 'sub-clinical neurosis', and again close to the one in three mark. Women of course had higher scores, the mean being 15 for the women and 13 for the men. Scores increased with advancing age, and indeed some such relation with age was found by several of the earlier investigators we have encountered before.

Are figures of this kind typical of modern Western culture, as is sometimes assumed, or would similar rates of incidence be found in non-Western cultures? The hypothesis that mental disorders are largely genetic in origin, even though environmental influences are also implicated, would suggest that more primitive cultures would also be found to have their fair share of neurotic upsets, although these might not be so easy to discover in the absence of hospital and other medical provision. A recent study was carried out in a group of three small villages in Southern India, Kota, with a population of about 9,000. The communities studied were Brahmins, mostly high-caste and landowners; Bants, who are mostly agriculturists; and Mogers, who are traditionally fishermen. The nearest mental hospital was 250 miles distant, the nearest trained psychiatrist 70 miles away. In all, 1,233 individuals were interviewed, and it was discovered that no less than 37 per cent admitted at least one psychiatric symptom. Such symptoms were commoner amongst females, and among the poorer members of the community. Not all those belonging to the one-third afflicted with some psychiatric symptom were of course seriously ill, or required hospitalization, but it is interesting that the figure should be so close to that found in eighteenth century or modern England, in spite of the tremendous cultural and other differences between these countries. At the lowest estimate, it was concluded that 6 per cent of those interviewed required urgent psychiatric help, suggesting that if these figures were typical (and in some ways Kota was better off than most Indian communities, assuming that this has something to do with mental health), then 18 million people in India needed psychiatric assistance and treatment, mainly of course for neurotic disorders. Other less systematic studies of primitive tribes, and also of more advanced African and Asian communities, have given similar figures; it is also noteworthy that symptoms typical of neurotic disorders in the West are found equally typical elsewhere. Neurosis is a world-wide problem, and its causation cannot be linked with advancing culture.

What can we conclude from all this evidence? M. Lader, who has made a careful study of the published accounts, puts it this way. 'Do ten million adults in Great Britain have symptoms of anxiety, insufficient to cause them to seek medical aid yet great enough to cause them discomfort, distress and suffering?' he asks, and answers: 'The evidence . . . is too consistent to ignore. What hospital psychiatrists are seeing is the tip of an iceberg; what general practitioners see is similarly but a fraction of human "dis-ease".' As Lader points out, the implications of the number of persons with subclinical anxiety or neurotic symptoms are frightening.

> The case load of psychiatrists and, particularly, of general practitioners could expand almost indefinitely. In the United Kingdom the average general practitioner would have about 500 subclinical anxious patients on his list, for whom he would be contractually obliged to provide treatment. If they all insisted on their rights and were each allocated only 15 minutes per week for a supportive psychotherapeutic interview, the general practitioner would be working 125 hours per week on this one condition. Patients are becoming more demanding and expect effective medical treatment not only for major acute illnesses but for minor chronic conditions as well. The potential for overloading the health services is only too plain to see.

Patients of this kind often receive sympathetic treatment, even though this cannot in the majority of cases be of a skilled psychiatric kind; most of the time the symptoms are treated with anxiety-allaying drugs, tranquillizers, and the like. The cost of these drugs to the National Health Service is in the neighbourhood of thirty million pounds per annum, and although these drugs are fairly effective and safe in use, they often give rise to long-term dependence. They certainly do not provide a cure; they are only a palliative.

Lader, like most psychiatrists, assumes that neurotic disorders are in some sense diseases, and hence a medical problem. This is one way of looking at the position; as we shall see, there are other ways. Neuroses and other mental disorders may be looked upon as moral problems; in catholic countries, at least, far more neurotics consult their priest than consult the psychiatrist. In the USA several studies have shown that only a small minority of neurotics go to see the psychiatrist; many more see ministers of religion, quacks, counsellors, favourite aunts, psychologists –

almost anybody but a medically qualified healer. The reason is only partly monetary; for most people medicine seems inappropriate to their troubles. In this they may very well be right. We shall see soon that neurotic disorders may with advantage be looked upon as learned reactions which can be unlearned; none of this involves medical factors, and it is doubtful if medical training is relevant to the appropriate treatment. What this is, again, we shall have to see later.

It is pretty clear that the group of 'neurotics' is not homogeneous. They can all be placed, with more or less confidence, along a continuum which may be labelled the 'diathesis-stress continuum'. Diathesis is simply a medical term for predisposition to develop a particular disorder; in other words, some people have such a strong genetic predisposition for emotional upsets, 'nerves', worries, anxieties, etc. that the slightest stress will set them off. They make up the 5 per cent or so of the population which shows lifelong anxiety of an almost entirely constitutional nature. Symptoms vary in kind and strength, but are rarely absent, and the prognosis is not good. At the other end of the continuum are people who are constitutionally normal, but have suffered overwhelmingly strong stress; the traumatic wartime neuroses are largely of this nature. Here prognosis is good. The great bulk of subclinical neurotics are between these extremes, showing both predisposition (diathesis) and stress. Actually the nature of the 'stress' involved is not at all clearly understood, and confidently proclaimed views on this subject are rarely backed up by factual and experimental material. Psychoanalytic speculations in particular are rife, but without empirical support. Lader suggests that 'probably, attitudes toward neurosis on the part of the general practitioner and of the general public are the most important factors in determining the incidence of overt neurosis. A kind, sympathetic doctor with time to listen will find many of his patients with a subclinical anxiety state developing overt symptoms.' This is a reasonable hypothesis, but again firm support is so far missing.

Summary

The reader could hardly be blamed if he felt that our knowledge of the nature and incidence of neurosis was remarkably lacking in substance and content. We cannot define neurosis unambiguously – indeed, we cannot for sure say whether there is such a thing or not. We do not know how many people are suffering from this possibly non-existent disease. We do not know that, if it existed, it could be considered a disease, in the medical meaning. If it were a disease, we would not know how to treat it, except through palliative drugs. In any case, whatever it is, it is pretty heterogeneous. Heredity seems to play a part, but so does the environment – if only we knew what aspects of the environment were involved! In any case, huge numbers of people seem to be afflicted by this undefinable 'disease', putting a great stress on the health services. The whole thing is paradoxical, frightening, and productive of a great deal of suffering. In this confusing situation, there are loud voices stridently proclaiming that they and they alone have the key, not only to the nature and cause of the disorder, but also to the cure. Unfortunately, these voices contradict each other; furthermore, they fail to produce any acceptable evidence in support of their claims. No wonder most people feel confused and frightened at the same time, and do not like even to mention the dread word, mental illness. Nevertheless, this is the situation. We must accept the facts as they are; can research throw any light on the causes and cures of neurosis?

2 Causes of Neurosis

Demonology and psychoanalysis

Until nearly the turn of this century, the most widespread and indeed almost universal theory of mental illness was in terms of demonic or satanic possession; a person behaving in a manner lacking insight (as does the psychotic) or counter to his own declared intentions and wishes (as does the neurotic) could only do so because he was possessed by an alien force. This force must clearly come from the evil one, being opposed to normal, God-fearing behaviour as demonstrated by normal, God-fearing people. This diagnosis of the cause equally indicated the cure — exorcism. If some little Satan or Beelzebub caused these distressing symptoms, then the priest, or the witchdoctor, or whoever, must use the powers of his religious office to drive out the devil. If in the course of these procedures the patient got damaged (often irretrievably) it mattered little; his immortal soul was at stake, and no consideration for his body was allowed to interfere.

It should not be imagined that these methods are necessarily useless and absurd, simply because they stem from an obviously erroneous notion of the cause of mental illness. Professor K. Jaspers, one of the most renowned of the great school of German psychiatrists in pre-Hitler days, stated explicitly that there was no doubt in his own mind that psychoanalysts, psychotherapists and other medical practitioners were decidedly inferior, as far as effectiveness of treatment went, to 'shamans, medicinemen, priests, religious leaders, saints and quacks of all sorts'. The reason, of course, was that for the believer the influence of a person of this kind is out of all proportion to the rational content of any message that passes between the two; suggestibility is raised to a point where startling mental and bodily phenomena become commonplace.

It would, indeed, be quite wrong to imagine that we must know the true cause of a disorder before we can treat it successfully. Historically, the discovery of the syndrome usually

37

precedes the discovery of the 'cause' of the disease – assuming for the moment that indeed there is a single cause, rather than a whole set of causal factors which work together to produce the 'disease'. Thus the Roman writer Celsus (25 BC – AD 50) already discusses tuberculosis in his book *De Medicina*, although the discovery of the tubercle bacillus did not take place until 1882. Nor did treatment always wait upon the discovery of the 'cause'. Aretaeus the Cappadocian, who lived in the third century AD, is credited with the advocacy of a milk diet in phthisis, to take but one example. In the eighteenth century the cause of the scurvy was not known, but fresh fruit juices were used to prevent its occurrence. Jenner did not know the cause of smallpox, nor why vaccination should afford protection against the disease. Thus lack of knowledge, and even the assumption of quite unreasonable 'causes', need not prevent us from arriving at remedies which may be quite effective. Exorcism probably worked quite well in certain cases, but the general lack of religious feeling at the present time makes it quite useless as a remedy for neurotic and other mental ills.

Satanic possession and exorcism were replaced as causal factors in the explanation of neurosis by psychoanalysis, and for the last fifty years it has been the theories of Freud and his followers which have held major sway over the minds of psychiatrists and psychologists alike. It would be quite inappropriate to go into these theories in any detail; only a very short and meagre account of the main outlines of these theories will be given, leading to a discussion of the methods of treatment based upon them. This may seem unfair, but many other accounts are available, and in any case, as we shall point out, these theories and methods are now only of historical interest. Briefly, then, Freud adopted a medical model according to which the 'symptoms' complained of by the patient were the outcome of the revival of certain 'complexes' which had been laid down in his extreme youth; treatment had to concern itself with these complexes, rather than with the symptoms. The prime and indeed universal complex was of course the Oedipus complex. According to this fable each boy falls in love with his mother, desires her sexually, but represses this desire because of fear of his father. The unconscious complex festers on and gives rise to symptoms when certain events in the life history of the patient weaken resistances or awaken the latent complex. Treatment consists essentially in endless talks during which the analyst tries to obtain some idea of the inner dynamics of the patient's life, through dream interpretation, through word association, or through apparently aimless chatter on the part of the patient who is exhorted to say anything that comes into his mind. The analyst then attempts to make the patient remember and integrate into his present life these memories of the situations which originated the complex — not only intellectually but also emotionally. This takes a long time (even assuming it can be done at all, and assuming that in fact there is anything at all to remember and integrate). Typically psychoanalysis still takes several years, with an hour a day spent five days a week with the analyst — at a cost (in America) of 50 dollars an hour, give or take a few dollars. A proper analysis is thus likely to cost around 50,000 dollars, assuming an average course of four years; some take less, but some take a good deal more, and analyses of twenty years' duration are not unheard of.

This very inadequate summary leaves out of account many interesting and indeed fascinating inmates of the Freudian menagerie. Thus we have a censor busily refusing to let turbulent ideas become conscious, although he occasionally nods at night time, and allows unholy thoughts to come out in disguise in our dreams. The trinity of the ego, the super-ego and the id make their appearance, and so do Eros and Thanatos, the love and death instincts. Freud rummaged through the whole of Greek mythology to name his many creations, but we must forbear to enter into these amazing and fabulous details. The jungle of the Unconscious is full of dangerous monsters, with only the ever-vigilant analyst as a protection for the unwary patient. The actual details of the story vary very much; different analysts have quite different tales to tell of their adventures in this land of mystery. Even the same teller often changes his mind; Freud's own account differs each time the tale is retold. Much of what Freud has to say is of course merely a repetition of other people's thoughts. Plato told the fable of the coachman who has to control his two horses, the good horse and the bad; the coachman is the ego, the good horse the super-ego, the bad horse the id. The main difference is that Plato knew he was telling a fable to illustrate a philosophical point; Freud was under the erroneous impression that he was constructing a scientific theory. Even the unconscious was not an invention of Freud's; at least two hundred other authors, from the most ancient times right up to his own, had preceded him in postulating something of the sort.

It may be useful to give readers at this point an example which will illustrate the sort of theories which Freudians put forward to explain certain neurotic symptoms, and to contrast this with a more scientific type of explanation. The example chosen is on purpose selected to be rather simple and unimportant; we shall deal with more complex cases later. However, the case of *enuresis nocturna,* or simple bed-wetting, is very instructive; it will demonstrate a number of interesting points which we shall later on embroider. The facts are quite simple; many children wet their beds at night, even at an age when the great majority of their brothers and sisters have ceased to do so. Why? And what can we do about it? Psychoanalysts regard enuresis with grave suspicion; as one of them has said, 'enuresis is always regarded in psychoanalysis as a symptom of a deeper underlying disorder'. According to this point of view, the clinician attaches fundamental causal importance to the deep-seated patterns of the child-parent relationships which are 'moulded from birth due to the complex interplay of unconscious forces from both sides'. Some of the specific theories embraced by analysts take the form of highly speculative interpretations based on psychoanalytical symbolism. For one analyst, for instance, enuresis 'represented a cooling of the penis, the fire on which was condemned by the super-ego'. For another, enuresis was an attempt to escape a masochistic situation and to expel outwards the destructive tendencies: the urine is seen as a corrosive fluid and the penis as a dangerous weapon. Yet another therapist suggested that usually enuresis expresses a demand for love, and might be a form of 'weeping through the bladder'.

There are too many different speculations of this kind among psychoanalytic writers to list them all; they can conveniently be grouped under three different headings. Some believe that enuresis is a substitute form of gratification of repressed genital sexuality — if I can't sleep with my mother, then I'll use my penis this way. Others regard enuresis as a direct manifestation of deep-seated anxieties and fears. Yet others interpret it as a disguised form of hostility towards parents or parent substitutes which the victim does not dare to express openly — if I can't attack you openly because you are stronger, then I'll annoy you this way! All these theories insist on the primacy of some psychological 'complex', and the secondary nature of the 'symptom'; concern is with the former, not the latter. Consequently, treatment is long drawn-out, involves searching examination of the patient's unconscious through dream interpretation, word-association, and other complex methods, and enters into consideration of many aspects of the child's personality apparently irrelevant to the simple act of bed-wetting. Does all this complex machinery produce an effect?

There is no doubt that children so treated over a number of years often do show an improvement, and quite a high proportion of them will emerge cured. But this is not a fair test. It is well known that most enuretic children remit spontaneously as they get older; that is, they get better even when not given any psychiatric or medical treatment at all. At the age of five, some 12 per cent of all children bed-wet, but at the age of twelve, say, only very few do; the rest have given it up without any treatment. Thus the therapist is on a good wicket, very much as is the physician who treats a common cold. Whatever he does, it is likely to improve, and the grateful patient will thank the doctor for his treatment, even though the cure might have been accomplished just as quickly without it. In order to prove the usefulness of his treatment, one would have to show that the treatment does better than no treatment. We need clinical trials in which patients are allocated at random to a treatment group, given psychoanalysis or whatever is alleged to 'cure' the patient, and a control group, given either no treatment or better still a 'placebo' treatment, some form of meaningless and certainly ineffective 'cure' that makes the patient imagine that something is being done for him when in fact he is simply receiving, say, a dummy pill made up of sugar and flour. Such a placebo treatment is important; suggestible patients may get better when the fact that they are being 'treated' impresses them so much that the suggestion works and makes them abandon their 'symptom'. Thus psychoanalysis might work, as compared with 'no treatment', simply because of some suggestion effect; this would be ruled out by having a plausible placebo treatment. Experiments have shown that the effectiveness of anti-pain pills and injections is about 50 per cent due to suggestion; in other words, placebo pills and injections, having no physiological effect whatever, are at least half as effective (and may be just as effective) as aspirin and morphine! Suggestibility is an important factor that should always be carefully controlled in experiments of this kind, particularly when the alleged effects are partly or wholly mental.

Does psychotherapy work when conditions are properly controlled in this fashion, when we are running our experimental group against a properly matched placebo or no-treatment group? The answer is not known; psychoanalysts and psychotherapists, here as in other more important areas, have completely neglected to back up their far-reaching claims with appropriate experiments or clinical trials. From such papers as have been published, and from what we know about the natural course of enuresis in children, we can construct some sort of an answer, although of course this is much less satisfactory a method than direct clinical comparison. Such an answer would be in the negative; children suffering from enuresis and treated by experienced psychoanalysts, or by psychotherapists using analytic concepts and methods, do not seem to get better any more quickly than do children not treated at all. It seems possible that compared with a placebo treatment group psychoanalysis would do even worse, but the data are not sufficient at the moment to make this assertion with any degree of confidence. However, no such proof is needed; let us merely note at this point that there is no published evidence to suggest that psychoanalysis cures or improves enuresis in children or adults. This must make one very suspicious of any claims for the correctness of the theory involved, both as regards the origin of the 'symptom' and as regards the method of treatment.

It is interesting to note that long before mediaeval demonology and Victorian psychoanalysis came into existence, there existed already the rudiments of the theory which was later to account for neurotic fears and anxieties in a much more economical and scientific fashion. These ancient theories were Greek in origin, but they were voiced in their most convincing form by Marcus Tullius Cicero, in his *Tuscularum Disputationum*. In the first place he points out that '*Ab earum rerum est absentium metus, quarum est aegritudo*': in neurotic disorders, anxiety is felt of things not present, the presence of which causes grief, or distress. This suggests immediately a learning process by means of which the distress properly associated with the 'thing present' (the unconditioned stimulus, in modern parlance) is evoked when the 'thing' is not present; that is, through a conditioned stimulus. Now if we can remove the distress reaction, then the neurotic anxiety also will be taken away: *'Sublata igitur aegritudine sublatus est metus.'* This of course suggests a method of extinction, whether through 'desensitization', or 'flooding', or 'modelling'.

Cicero finally caps his account by appealing to individual differences: *'At qui in quem cadit aegritudo, in eundem timor; quarum enim rerum praesentia sumus in aegritudine, eadem impendentes et venientes timemus.'* Translated freely, this states that the man who is easily distressed is also an ˍasy prey to anxiety or fear. For when stimuli cause distress by their presence, we are also afraid of the menace of their approach. In other words, people who have strong fear reactions to actual dangers and stressful situations also show strong learned anxieties in the absence of these stimuli. We cannot follow Cicero into the details of his discussion, but the elements of our modern way of looking at neurosis are certainly contained in his account.

Biological factors

Is there an alternative to psychoanalysis? There is indeed, and it is typical of the approach advocated in this book. The view taken by exponents of this alternative view is that in the majority of cases enuresis may be regarded simply as the failure to acquire a habit. This 'habit deficiency' is due to faulty habit training of some kind. Ordinary continence training teaches the child to respond to bladder stimulation by awakening. The child thus learns to substitute going to the toilet (or using his pot) for bedwetting; when this learning fails, enuresis is the result. A thorough investigation has shown that, although there is sometimes something physically wrong with the urinary system, bed-wetting is a habit condition in nine cases out of ten. A somewhat different view is taken by those who believe that simple enuresis is a continuation into childhood of the automatic bladder reflexes of infancy, whereas in the case of more complicated types of enuresis the child has acquired habits of urinating during sleep in response to specific environmental conditions. Both types of enuresis are ascribed to faulty training procedures.

There are two major 'causes' of this alleged habit deficiency, both of which may of course be active in combination to produce the effect. One is faulty training, or insufficient training, or some similar environmental cause; the other is lack of trainability on the part of the child. The latter condition might be simply due to the fact that the child is sleeping unusually deeply and hence does not wake up to the prompting of the full bladder; or it could be that he is constitutionally predisposed to have difficulties in making the necessary neural connections between the stimulus (the full bladder) and the response (waking up). Both conditions apparently play a part, with extraverted children having greater difficulties than introverted ones. We shall see later on why this should be so, but here we shall not go into the theory of the genesis of enuresis any further, but look rather at the suggested methods of treatment which follow from such a model.

The hypothesis states that there is a failure on the part of the child to connect the stimulus and the response; the treatment should therefore consist in creating conditions which would lead to such a connection being made. The first to suggest a practical method for this was an English pediatrician, Dr J. Nye, who outlined his proposed treatment thus in 1830:

Attach one pole of an electric battery to a moist sponge or a metallic plate fastened between the shoulders of the patient and the other to a dry sponge attached to the *meatus urinarius* [the urinary outlet]. When this has been done and arranged so as not to annoy the patient, let him be put to bed and the circuit of the bed completed. The sound of the battery will soon lull the patient to sleep. While the sponge is dry, no electricity passes through the body of the patient, and his slumber is undisturbed, but the moment the patient begins to urinate, the sponge is moistened and becomes a conductor of electricity. The circuit is completed through the body of the patient and he or she is at once aroused, awakened and caught in the very act and thus caveat is entered by the will as well as by the electricity against further proceeding at least for this time. A repetition of a like experience a sufficient number of times ought, I am inclined to think, to cure the patient, but since this suggestion has occurred to me I have not had the opportunity of putting it to the test of practical experiment and submit it to the consideration of the profession for what it is worth.

We now know that the method would have worked very well indeed.

What is taking place in the proposed set-up is a process of Pavlovian conditioning. Pavlov's original experiment is well enough known to demand little by way of explanation. He demonstrated that dogs would not salivate to the sound of a bell, but would salivate to the sight of food. He would then pair the two stimuli (bell—food) a number of times, until finally the bell (the so-called conditioned stimulus or CS) would produce copious salivation even in the absence of the food (the unconditioned stimulus or US). In the set-up described above the enlarged bladder would constitute the CS and the tingling sensation produced by the electric circuit, waking the patient up, the US; after a few repetitions, the CS would produce the effect previously only produced by the US — wake up the patient before he wet his bed. Thus the habit deficiency is cured by supplementing the usual training procedures in this specific manner. A method similar to that suggested by Nye has been used very successfully in Australia, but the most widely used method, which originated in Germany at the turn of the century, uses instead a blanket interleaved between two porous metal plates; these plates are connected in series with a battery and a bell. The dry blanket acts as an insulator; once the child begins to wet the blanket the saline urine begins to act as an electrolyte and a connection is made between the metal plates. This completes the circuit, and the bell rings and wakes up the child — and causes him reflexly to inhibit the act of urination. This method is now very widely used in child guidance clinics all over the world; it is completely safe and has been found acceptable to parents and children alike. Does it work?

Figure 1 shows the results of applying three different treatments to groups of enuretics. The first of these was a placebo treatment, a dummy treatment not meant to have any effect other than to provide a control for suggestibility, and the illusion of having been helped. It will be seen that over the period of six weeks that the test lasted, there was no improvement of any kind in the patients making up this group. The two other groups received the 'bell-and-blanket' treatment, but with one impor-

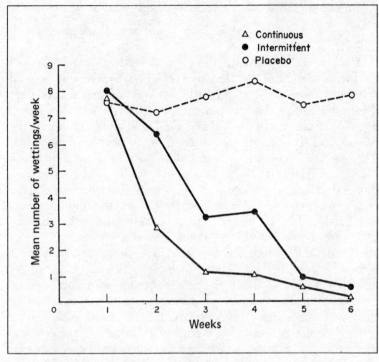

FIGURE 1
The effects of different methods of treatment on
nocturnal enuresis.

tant difference. One group had the instrument connected up each
time; the other only had it connected up two times out of three,
so that on one occasion in three the patient would not have the
pairing of bladder enlargement and bell-awakening. The former
method is called *continuous reinforcement*, the latter *intermittent reinforcement*, meaning that the pairing between CS and US is
effected continually or intermittently. The reason for this distinction will become apparent very soon; for the moment note simply that under both conditions the mean number of wettings per
week sinks for both groups from an average of eight to an
average of less than one – meaning of course that the majority of
the children were completely cured. Intermittent reinforcement
may seem a little less efficacious, which is hardly surprising, but it

gets down to pretty much the same degree of amelioration or cure.

We thus find this method to be simple, quick, and labour-saving. The treatment is done at home, by the parents, and does not require the services of a psychologist or psychiatrist except at the beginning, to inaugurate the treatment, and occasionally during its course to keep track of what is happening. It provides definitive evidence of effectiveness (this is of course not the only such study; there are very many others which demonstrate the same point). Last but not least, the treatment has 'face validity'; in other words, the parent and the child immediately understand its rationale, and find no difficulty in agreeing to cooperate and work the system. These are important advances.

The experiment whose results are depicted in Figure 1 may now be used to decide between the two theories we are concerned with, the psychoanalytic and the behavioural. Both theories make predictions and in so far as these are in conflict the experiment may serve to tell us which theory is right – or rather, which theory is better in agreement with the facts. (In science, no theory can ever be called 'right'; it may work today, but tomorrow another fact may appear which cannot be understood in terms of our theory.) Let us then consider the predictions made by the two theories, and let us also consider some further facts produced by the experiment but not discussed so far.

In the first place, psychoanalysts would not have predicted that the treatment would actually work. At best they might have said that in a few isolated cases such purely 'symptomatic' treatment could be successful for a limited period. Behavioural scientists, on the other hand, could and did predict success; as we have seen, some 150 years ago this prediction was already made. On this point, then, we must score a 'plus' for the behavioural theory, and a 'minus' for the psychoanalytic one.

The children have nearly all learned the desired behaviour; are they likely to relapse? Learning theory would say that there was a fair chance that many of them would relapse. The reason is simply that all conditioned responses are subject to extinction. We shall discuss extinction in some detail later (because it is a very important concept in the elimination of neurotic disorders) but here let us simply note that conditioned responses are produced by pairing the CS and the US; when they are later uncoupled and the CS is produced by itself, without the US, then there is a tendency for the link to be broken and extinction to take place. Such extinction would appear in the form of a relapse, and such relapses do in fact occur in a fair number of patients. Psychoanalysts would have to predict that relapses should occur in all the children successfully treated. If the disorder is due to the nervous 'complexes' Freudians allege to be responsible, then only the elimination of these complexes can permanently cure the child; anything else is purely symptomatic, and is bound to lead to relapse. This is clearly untrue for the majority of children. The facts bear out the prediction made from the behavioural theory, not that made from the psychoanalytic one.

Psychoanalysts have an alternative hypothesis. They say that instead of a relapse the patient may show 'symptom substitution'; in other words, if the complex is not eradicated, then either the same symptom reappears after purely symptomatic treatment (relapse) or else another symptom altogether may appear (symptom substitution). In the case of enuresis they have often predicted that the anxiety so often noted in enuretic children might get much worse, even though the actual enuresis might not reappear. This prediction is of course derived from the fact that psychoanalysts believe that enuresis is produced as the result of serious anxiety already present in the child, producing the symptom of enuresis as an expression of that anxiety. Behavioural scientists hold the opposite view; they believe that the anxiety is produced by the after-effects of the enuresis, the censure to which this leads, the scolding, the difficulties with a child's peers, and so on. Eliminate the enuresis and the anxiety should also disappear. The facts support the latter hypothesis; many therapists have looked for substitute symptoms, particularly increased anxiety, but have uniformly failed to find any such effects. Here again, psychoanalysis scores a 'minus', behavioural treatment a 'plus'.

If the relapses observed in these children are due to insufficient learning, then we should be able to deduce from learning theory methods of avoiding the majority of these relapses. This can indeed be done. One such method is 'overlearning'. Extinction takes place, in part, because the new habit has not been established strongly enough; the difficulty is to establish it more strongly. When you condition a dog to salivate to the sound of a bell, you can pair the bell and the food hundreds and indeed thousands of times; there is no limit. You can go on long after the link has been established very securely. In the case of enuresis you cannot do this; once the enuretic has ceased to wet the bed, you cannot link the CS and the US, simply because there is no more US! You can do two things, however, to redress the balance. If a child relapses, you can retrain him by producing a few bell-and-blanket CS – US connections; this is usually enough to make the cure permanent. Or you can make the child drink a lot of water before retiring; although he is cured as far as the ordinary amount of water intake is concerned, this additional intake puts a further strain on his bladder and he is likely to revert to bed-wetting. Thus now you can give him some further training, and having 'overlearned' the habit he is much less likely to relapse. Both these methods have been shown to work very well, and thus score another 'plus' for behavioural therapy.

However, much of what we have said so far may sound less than impressive because it is really not far removed from common sense – the facts unearthed may be interesting, but they are not exactly surprising. There is, however, one prediction which would not be made on common sense grounds, and it is this prediction which was tested in our experiment by having one group with continuous and another with intermittent reinforcement. Learning theory predicts, and experiment has verified, that extinction is much slower and less powerful after intermittent than after continuous reinforcement. If relapses are in fact just examples of the extinction of a conditioned response, then we would expect relapse of our enuretic children to be less frequent in the group where conditioning was intermittent, as compared with the group where it was continuous. This is precisely what was found; there was a significant difference in frequency of relapse, in the predicted direction. This is a very unlikely thing to happen by chance; it suggests that the theory on which this treatment is based is largely along the right lines. Another + then, for the behavioural therapy.

The bell-and-blanket method is now very widely used in child guidance clinics and elsewhere, and hardly anyone would nowadays even think of using psychoanalysis for the treatment of enuresis. However, it may be useful to remember some of the difficulties that arose when the behavioural methods of treatment were first mooted, around the time of the Second World War.

The incidents to be related happened to me personally, and are literally true in every particular; they may illustrate the sort of distortions and refusals which a new theory may have to suffer before it is widely accepted. When I tried to get the consultant in charge of the Children's Department in the Hospital where I was working to introduce the bell-and-blanket method on an experimental basis, he swore that as long as he was alive no child under his care would be exposed to this invention of the devil; psychotherapy was the only method that was to be used, and he would refuse even to read the evidence on the basis of which I was suggesting the introduction of this evil machine! (No need to emphasize that the record of treatment for enuresis was distinctly poor in this Department. Indeed, we had to wait until his death before his successors used the bell-and-blanket, only to find, of course, that it was much the treatment of choice for enuresis.

When I published some tentative suggestions as to the use of this new method, a well-known psychoanalyst fulminated in the popular press about this sadist who was intent on giving electric shocks to the penises of young boys! I tried to point out that the method did not involve any sort of shock at all, but to no avail; the label of 'sadist' stuck for a long time. Some psychoanalysts even nowadays still have some very curious ideas about the methods used by behavioural scientists!

Around the same time, I received a letter from an American woman who had read some of my writings and asked me for information of how to get a bell-and-blanket apparatus. She had got in touch with a psychiatric hospital in her home town, but had been brushed off with a letter which she enclosed. What this letter stated had such a classical simplicity and charm that it may repay summarising. According to the psychiatrist in charge of the children's clinic, there was no such method as that recommended by me. If there was such a method, it could not possibly work. And if it did work he was damned if he was going to help anybody to find out about it. This was the atmosphere in which behavioural methods grew up, and the misconceptions rife then can still be found in many quarters.

Anxiety and conditioning

Modern theories of neurosis are based on a fundamental fact of biological reality and evolutionary progress, namely the fact that mankind has evolved through several stages, from reptilian to mammalian, and that our brain still bears the traces of this evolution. Just as Schliemann, digging up the ancient city of Troy, found that several cities had been built on top of each other on the site, so also in our brain do we find that several layers of evolutionary development are superimposed on each other. We like to think of ourselves in terms of *homo sapiens*, rational man, but that part of our brain which subserves rational thinking, the bulging grey matter underneath our skull, is carefully wrapped around more ancient, non-rational portions of our brain which still determine much of what we do, what we aim at and what we seek to achieve. It is these ancient relics of our past, millions of years ago, which come to plague us in the form of neurotic symptoms.

We might say that we suffer from a generation gap on a truly gigantic scale, a generation gap not on an ontogenetic scale, like that due to our growing older, and not maintaining contact with the younger people in our society, but rather on a phylogenetic scale, that is, related to our whole evolutionary development. Paul MacLean, chief of the Laboratory of Brain Evolution and Behaviour at the National Institute of Mental Health in the USA, has put it very clearly:

In evolution the primate forebrain expands along the lines of three basic patterns characterized as reptilian, paleomammalian, and neo-mammalian. The result is the remarkable linkage of three brain types which are radically different in structure and chemistry, and which, in an evolutionary sense, are countless generations apart. We possess, so to speak, a hierarchy of three-brains-in-one — a triune brain. Or, stated another way, we have a linkage of three biocomputers, each with its own special kind of intelligence, sense of time, memory, motor, and other functions. Although my proposed scheme for subdividing the brain may seem simplistic, the fact remains that the three basic formations are there for anyone to see, and, thanks to improved anatomical, chemical, and physiological techniques, stand out in clearer detail than ever before. It should be emphasized, although they are separate, they are capable of functioning somewhat independently.

What do these three 'brains' do that sets them apart from each other? According to MacLean, the reptilian brain is basic for such genetically constituted behaviour as selecting home site, establishing and defending territory, hunting, homing, mating, forming social hierarchies and the like. In humans especially, he believes that the reptilian brain is involved with compulsive, repetitious, ritualistic, deceptive, and imitative forms of behaviour. Essentially, much of our more primitive, instinctive behaviour is built on these physiological foundations, reaching back through 250 million years of history, to the age of the reptiles. As MacLean points out,

> it is traditional to belittle the role of instincts in human behaviour, but how should we categorize those actions that stem from a predisposition to compulsive and ritualistic behaviour; a proclivity to prejudice and deception; a propensity to seek and follow precedent as in legal and other matters; and a natural tendency to imitation? All these propensities have survival value, but they are double-edged and can cut both ways.

Reptiles have only a rudimentary cortex, and in the transition to mammals it is thought that this was expanded and elaborated, providing the animal with a better means for viewing the environment and learning to survive. In both lower and higher mammals the old cortex occupies a large convolution (the limbic lobe) which surrounds the brain stem. This primitive limbic cortex is concerned with emotional behaviour such as is observed in fear and anger, and with feeding, fighting, and self-protection. Genital and other forms of sexual behaviour have also recently been found related to this paleomammalian brain (paleo = ancient), suggesting that it is concerned with expressive and feeling states which promote the procreation of the species. There are also suggestions that this system may be concerned fundamentally with the development of a feeling of individuality and personal identity. These are all important functions, but they are clearly still differentiated from cognitive behaviour, inductive and deductive reasoning, and other peculiarly human behaviour patterns.

Compared with the limbic cortex, the new cortex is like an

expanding numerator. It mushrooms late in evolution, culminating in man to become the brain of reading, writing, and arithmetic. Mother of invention and father of abstract thought, it promotes the preservation and procreation of ideas.

The limbic system, that part of the old or paleomammalian brain which is responsible for emotional arousal and the expression and coordination of emotion, probably reacts directly only to such immediate sensory inputs as pain and pleasure. However, an animal which was incapable of anticipating these direct and immediate consequences of its actions would be severely handicapped; it clearly needs some form of signalling system which provides it with preliminary warning of forthcoming events likely to impinge upon it and to have rewarding or punishing consequences. Such a system is provided by Pavlov's conditioning mechanism; it is probably most useful to look upon conditioning in the light of evolutionary development as a rather elementary mechanism for the anticipation of future events on a simple probability basis. As we shall see, Pavlov also recognizes the existence of a second signalling system, namely rational, cognitive thought mediated through the neocortex; this is clearly superior in effectiveness to conditioning, and perhaps should take its place were we really designed by some omnipotent deity *de novo*. However, no such entirely new designs exist in nature; we all bear the traces of our ancestry, and in the case of conditioning, humans as well as animals, from the lowest to the highest, still carry with them the imprint of this ancient, primitive system of anticipation which undoubtedly was extremely useful once, but which now is often superfluous and may interfere disastrously with the second signalling system. The modern theory of neurosis essentially maintains that neurotic problems and symptoms arise when there is a conflict between the messages received from the primitive conditioning system and those received from the more appropriate but less powerful second signalling system. The explanation of the neurotic paradox, in a nutshell, is that those actions which we call 'neurotic' are usually if not always provoked by the activity of the paleocortical mechanisms, particularly the limbic system, activated by a process of conditioning. The rational, conscious mind can recognize the inappropriate nature of these feelings (anxiety, fear, depression) but is powerless to override the more primitive system.

Some modern psychologists assert that 'conditioning theories are old-fashioned' and that 'cognitive' theories have taken their place. If what is meant is that human behaviour cannot be explained by conditioning mechanisms alone (or for that matter animal behaviour) then this assertion is undoubtedly true. After all, Pavlov himself stressed the importance of the second signalling system (which was his term for what nowadays would be called 'cognitive processes'); he would be the last person to deny its importance, particularly for human beings. But this does not mean that there is no such mechanism as primitive conditioning, or that this process may not powerfully determine the direction of our emotions. The evidence for some such process as that described by Pavlov is so overwhelming that it is difficult to see how anyone familiar with the literature can have any possible doubts on this score. To deny the importance of primitive conditioning, even in human beings, is as unscientific as to exaggerate it; what is needed is a proper appraisal of its place in the lives of humans and lower animals.

Let us look at a typical psychological experiment to illustrate some of these points. The experiment is conducted in what is known as a 'shuttle-box'. Usually the experimental animals are rats, but mostly it is preferable to work with dogs, so let us imagine that we are dealing with laboratory dogs in our experiment. The 'box' is constructed in such a way that we have two halves, separated by a hurdle; the dogs can easily jump over this hurdle to get from one side of the box to the other (i.e. 'shuttle' to and fro). Each side has a floor made of metal rods; these can be electrified separately, so as to give the dog an electric shock to his feet when he is on one side or the other. This shock is the unconditioned stimulus; it produces pain and leads the dog to jump over the hurdle into the other side of the box, which is left unelectrified. If we now introduce a signal to tell the dog that a shock is coming, he soon learns to jump at the signal, thus avoiding the shock. The usual signal is a blinking light, but of course any visual or auditory signal would do equally well. This signal is the conditioned stimulus; by itself it has no effect on the behaviour of the dog before it is paired with the shock. But once we let the light precede the shock a number of times by a few seconds, the conditioning process allows the animal to anticipate the shock, and he begins to jump to the light, thus avoiding the shock. (The phrase 'jump to the light' may be misleading; it means 'jump at the bidding of the light', not 'in the direction of the light'. The light is in fact suspended over the hurdle, and indicates 'danger' in either of the two chambers which make up the apparatus.)

This, then, is a typical paradigm of conditioning: the conditioned stimulus takes over the function of the unconditioned stimulus and allows the animal to *avoid* the noxious experience of the shock.

How does this process work? Clearly anxiety/fear is involved, because we can detect fearful behaviour in the dog when the conditioned stimulus appears – the dog yowls, urinates, runs about, and gives all the appearance of being afraid. Furthermore, we can measure psycho-physiological indices of fear, such as increased heart rate and faster breathing. One possibility is that what is conditioned is the emotional effect of the shock; by pairing light and shock, the light acquires the potency of producing fear/anxiety in the dog, and the dog reacts to this as he does to the shock, by jumping. In this way he assuages the fear/anxiety; it is reduced because experience has shown him that after the jump he is safe. Thus jumping behaviour is rewarded (by a decrease in anxiety) and he continues to jump to the light without ever again experiencing the shock. We may then say that anxiety is the mediating link in his behaviour, just as we shall see it is in human neurotic behaviour.

Actually the dog's behaviour so far is of course not neurotic, but perfectly reasonable. Using the primitive mechanism of the conditioned reflex the dog has learned to avoid the painful consequences of being shocked. However, he is not behaving in a rational manner, as can be shown quite simply by turning off the current altogether, so that the dog cannot be shocked any more, even if he refuses to jump to the light. Now, with the shock no longer a threat, it would be sensible to stop jumping, but the experimental animals continue to jump to the light; hundreds of trials fail to make them desist. This comes close to human phobic or obsessional behaviour, although of course the similarity must not be pressed too far. We can now give one more turn to the screw; let us actually *punish* the animal for jumping to the light. This can be done by connecting up the electricity again to the grid, but this time in such a manner that, when the light goes on, the side on which the dog is standing is safe, while that to which he jumps is electrified. Thus the conditioned stimulus is now connected up the wrong way; it should signal safety on the side where the dog is, and danger on the other side. In spite of this the dog will continue to jump, even though each time he is punished by a painful shock. This is an even more precise replica of human neurotic behaviour; mal-adaptive, self-punishing behaviour which has effects contrary to those sought by the organism.

There are other similarities with human neurosis. At first the dogs show signs of fear when the conditioned stimulus comes on, but once they have mastered the art of *avoiding* the shock through jumping to the light, they show little emotional reaction: they simply jump, without any indication of fear or anxiety. In a similar manner does the human obsessive-compulsive neurotic, afraid of contamination, show no fear or anxiety, even after getting dirty, as long as he is allowed to follow his washing and cleaning ritual. Anxiety only arises if man or dog is prevented from performing the conditioned act.

Why does the dog fail to learn that he need not jump any more, although it is perfectly safe to remain in his quarters, and even though he is actually incurring the penalty of being shocked through his jumping, instead of avoiding it? Possibly the answer lies in a fairly well supported general psychological law, which says, in brief, that $P = H \times D$; in other words, performance or behaviour is a multiplicative function of habit and drive. The habit in this case is the conditioned response of jumping; this is multiplied by the amount of drive or motivation spurring the animal on. Now the shock into which he jumps raises his fear/anxiety considerably, and this fear acts as a drive, thus multiplying with the habit of jumping and therefore making this particular performance even more an invariable consequence of the conditioned stimulus appearing. This is an important generalization which we shall encounter again in connection with the treatment of human neuroses; in order to get rid of the noisome neurotic habit we may have to reduce the amount of anxiety present to a tolerable level, thus also lowering the strength and likelihood of the performance of the neurotic act. This is one of the bases of the type of treatment we shall encounter under the name of 'desensitization'.

Another method would appear to proceed in exactly the opposite direction; this is the so-called method of 'response prevention' or 'flooding'; when used with human patients it is also sometimes known as 'catharsis' or 'implosion'. There is one sure way in which we can cure our dogs of their 'neurotic' behaviour; we can prevent their acting in this manner by increasing the height of the hurdle to such an extent that the dog can't jump over it when the light comes on. This produces a terrible excess of fear in the animal (hence the term 'flooding' – the animal is flooded by fear and anxiety). He runs around his side of the cage, yapping and howling; he attempts vainly to jump across to the other side; he may go through a veritable paroxysm of fear. But such outbursts do not last too long; after a while the dog calms down, and finally his emotion is all spent and he lies down quietly. Only a few such experiences of 'response prevention' are needed to cure him of his 'neurosis'; from then on he will no longer jump to the light, but disregard it completely. As we shall see later on, the method works just as well with human neurotics, although usually rather more time is required.

One further analogy exists between the behaviour of the dog, jumping even though this is clearly against his best interests, and the human neurotic, also acting in a manner prejudicial to his own advantage. Both fail to carry out what is sometimes called by psychiatrists 'reality testing'. Neurotics often state that they are afraid of certain animals, or people, or situations; they consequently avoid these animals, or people, or situations. Now in the past these stimuli (animals, people, situations) may have become conditioned stimuli for fear/anxiety reactions, through being associated with an unconditioned painful experience; the fact is, however, that this association was usually a fortuitous one and probably does not exist any longer. If only the neurotic could bring himself to experience the presence of the conditioned stimulus – the feared animal, person, or situation – he would soon discover that no terrible or painful consequences followed this exposure; by thus 'reality testing' he might discover (or rather, his limbic system might discover; his cortex is usually quite aware of it) that 'where hopes are dupes, fears may be liars' – in other words, that these conditioned stimuli are perfectly harmless. The dog, too, fails to 'reality test'; he jumps, instead of occasionally waiting to see if shock still follows light, and thus fails to discover that it would be perfectly safe to remain in his part of the shuttle-box. Response-prevention forces neurotic and dog to reality-test, and thus forces them into normal, non-neurotic behaviour.

Attentive readers will have noted an important difference between this experiment and the prototype of Pavlovian conditioning, namely the bell-saliva type of experiment. In that experiment, if the bell continues to be sounded without being followed by food, this produces extinction. That is one of the great laws discovered by Pavlov. Conditioned stimuli which are presented to the organism without being followed at some stage by unconditioned stimuli lead to extinction. In accordance with this law, ringing the bell, however closely it has been linked with salivation in the past, will produce a final cessation of salivation if it is rung frequently enough without the reinforcement of the food being added at some stage. Food does not *always* have to accompany the bell; the conditioned response can be maintained quite well if reinforcement is only given on two out of three occasions. Such partial reinforcement, as we have already seen in the case of the bell-and-blanket cure for enuresis, can be quite effective, and may in fact make for less marked extinction when reinforcement is completely withdrawn.

Now the case of the dogs in the light-shock situation is quite different. When the bell is not followed by food, there is no question of the dog's not knowing it, whereas in the shock experiment there is a complicating factor: the dog jumps to reduce or avoid anxiety, and by doing so protects the conditioned response (the anxiety) from extinction. In other words, this prevents the reality testing, which alone could produce extinction, from taking place. This great difference is probably parallel with the other major difference between the two experiments, which is that the unconditioned stimulus is noxious, painful or negatively reinforcing in the case of the shock, but nutritive, rewarding or positively reinforcing in the case of the food. We shall return to this distinction later on.

This type of experiment, dealt with at some length, is not the only animal analogue of human neurosis; there are many more. Pavlov, as usual, was the first to investigate this field. He conditioned dogs to salivate to a circle presented to them black on a white background. This may be called S+, the stimulus which received positive reinforcement. He also conditioned them *not* to salivate to an ellipse; this may be called S–, the stimulus which failed to get any positive reinforcement. (Actually at first, having become conditioned to salivate to the circle, the dogs also salivated to the ellipse; this is called *stimulus generalization*. Dogs, and humans, become conditioned not only to the actual stimulus which is paired with the unconditioned stimulus, but also to other stimuli which are in some way similar to the conditioned stimulus. Thus the ellipse, also drawn black on a white background, was sufficiently similar to the circle for the dogs to become conditioned to salivate to it also, although not as copiously; they had to become conditioned not to salivate to the ellipse, through repeated association between ellipse and no food.)

Having established this discrimination between circle and ellipse in the dogs, Pavlov went on to present them with ellipses which grew more and more circular, until the point was reached where the dogs could no longer distinguish between the two. At this point they had what might by analogy be called a nervous breakdown – they tore at their harness, refused to go into the experimental chamber, showed paradoxical reactions (salivating to the ellipse, but not to the circle), showed very strong emotional reaction, etc. Pavlov interpreted this behaviour in terms of conflict – he had set up an inescapable conflict in the animals between responding and not responding to stimuli which they could not properly distinguish, and this conflict, like the analogous but more serious conflicts to which human beings are exposed, produced a neurotic breakdown.

J. H. Masserman, a well-known psychiatrist, used another type of conflict to produce breakdown in cats. He taught them to lift the lid of a box with their noses in order to get food, which was put inside the box. He then arranged things in such a way that when they tried to open the lid, a strong blast of air was blown in their faces; this produced a strong conflict (avoiding the blast or trying to get the food) and the animals accordingly showed much fear and unease in approaching the box. Actually, like all analogue experiments, there is much uncertainty about the correct interpretation. We need not postulate any conflict in this situation at all, but merely note that having been 'punished' in this situation (through having air blown at them) the cats conditioned fear responses to the box and avoided it later on.

There would be little point in further detailing the many animal experiments which have been done in this field, or arguing about their interpretation. Suffice it to say that much knowledge about the conditioning process, about extinction, about generalization and other features of conditioning has been acquired along these lines, and that in particular our knowledge about fear/anxiety responses and their fate over time has been greatly increased by these experiments. Obviously this knowledge cannot immediately and directly be applied to human beings; humans are much more complex than animals such as dogs and cats. They possess a second signalling system, aided by language, which far surpasses anything other animals can show; and they are influenced by cultural and other factors which play no part in animal groups. But we may extract suggestions from this animal work, and try to adapt findings from animals to humans. ·The final and ultimate arbiter of our success must of course always be direct work with humans. Let me here anticipate later chapters by stating, quite unambiguously, that on the whole such application has been successful beyond what most psychologists would have hoped or expected.

3 A Theory of Neurosis

Watson's conditioning model

The theory here to be presented is an elaboration and amplification of a model originally suggested by J. B. Watson, the founder of behaviourism and one of the most original of the great American psychologists in the first two decades of this century. As he once put it, 'psychology as the behaviourist views it is a purely objective experimental branch of natural science. Its theoretical goal is the prediction and control of behaviour.' This of course is exactly what the psychiatrist and the clinical psychologist are trying to do – predict and control neurotic behaviour, and attempt to direct it in a direction more acceptable to the patient. Watson's contribution to this end has been extremely important, although the form his presentation took was rather unorthodox. Instead of elaborating his theory in detail, with copious references to the experimental literature, and then attempting to verify predictions derived from the theory, he published only a single case history, that of the famous 'little Albert', which he used to illustrate his theory. The theory itself is not worked out in detail but has to be more or less reconstructed from the bits and pieces strewn around this one case history. The paper itself, only ten pages long, was published jointly with Rosalie Rayner, his student and later his wife, as well as the cause of his much-publicized divorce and ultimate banishment from academic life by the Victorian conscience of an enraged university administration. (He went on to become a millionaire by using his psychological gifts in advertising – a great loss to psychology, but a gain to advertising!)

The reader should be warned that Watson's theory is overly simplistic, wrong in important aspects, and completely unacceptable both to experimental psychologists and to clinicians and psychiatrists. The case of little Albert, by being so clear-cut and so straightforward, has attracted a great deal of attention and has helped to paper over the very real difficulties which any con-

61

ditioning theory of neurosis (and in particular Watson's theory itself) has to face. Because Watson and Rayner present such an appealing case, relevant criticisms have not always been heard with enough diligence; in writing for the lay reader, in particular, many psychologists have failed to go into sufficient detail about the difficulties raised by the application of Watson's theory to adult human neuroses.

Why, the reader may wonder, should he be exposed to a theory both simplistic and essentially wrong? The answer is that often in science wrong theories point the way to real advances. As long as they are wrong in ways that can be corrected without abandoning the essential basis of the theory, so long will they remain scientifically important and fruitful. As an example, consider John Dalton, the originator of the modern atomic theory. All that Dalton said about atoms — apart from the bare fact of their existence, which was not novel — was wrong. They are not indivisible nor of unique weight, they need not obey the laws of definite or multiple proportions, and anyway his values for relative atomic weights and molecular constitutions were for the most part incorrect. Yet, for all that, he more than any other single individual was the man to set modern chemistry on its feet. For in devising a general scientific theory, the important thing is not to be right — such a thing in any final and absolute sense is beyond the bounds of mortal ambition. The important thing is to have the right idea, the fruitful notion which will enable scientists to pursue new paths, gather new insights, develop new territory — even if in doing so they succeed in demonstrating that many or even most of your original hypotheses were wrong. In the same way the importance of Watson's new idea lay not in the details but in the direction in which he pointed. He suggested an alternative to the sterile and unfruitful subjective psychoanalytical approach, and with all the errors and inadequacies his theory contains, it nevertheless marks the turning point in the history of neurosis where science took over. His theory was incorrect, but it was scientific in the sense that it was testable; no previous theory of neurosis had had that advantage. Future generations could build on what he had laid down, rejecting that which did not fit, retaining that which did. Hence this account, like all future ones, must begin with a consideration of his work.

Watson and Rayner begin their account by referring back to a theory previously advanced by Watson to the effect that in infancy the original emotional reaction patterns are few, consisting in the main of fear, rage and love. They go on to argue that 'there must be some simple method by means of which the range of stimuli which can call out these emotions and their compounds is greatly increased. Otherwise, complexity and adult response could not be accounted for.' They next advance the view that this range is increased by means of conditioning reflex activity, and they suggest that the early home life of a child furnishes a laboratory situation for establishing conditioned emotional responses. The article itself deals with an experimental test of this hypothesis, using only one child, Albert B. Albert was a normal healthy child who was tested at the age of approximately nine months. As the first step in the experiment

> the infant was confronted suddenly and for the first time successively with a white rat, a rabbit, a dog, a monkey, masks with and without hair, cotton wool, burning newspapers, etc. A permanent record of Albert's reactions to these objects and situations has been preserved in a motion picture study. Manipulation was the most usual reaction called out. *At no time did this infant ever show fear in any situation.* These experimental records were confirmed by the casual observations of the mother and the hospital attendants. No one had ever seen him in a state of fear and rage. The infant practically never cried.

White rats that were later to serve as conditioned stimuli thus produced no fear response of any kind. Looking for an unconditioned stimulus that would do so, Watson used a loud sound made by striking a hammer upon a suspended steel bar. This was done several times and on the third stimulation the child broke into a sudden crying fit. 'This is the first time an emotional situation in the laboratory has produced any fear or even crying in Albert.'

At the age of eleven months the experimenters began to condition a fear response to the rat by pairing the sight of the animal with the fear-producing sound of the hammer striking the metal bar. The process is described in detail by the authors, and after a number of repetitions, there is the following entry in their records. '*Rat alone. The instant the rat was shown the baby began to cry. Almost instantly he turned sharply to the left, fell over on left side, raised himself on all fours and began to crawl away so rapidly that he was caught with difficulty before reaching the edge of the table.'* Watson and Rayner go on to say 'this was as convincing a case of a completely conditioned fear response as could have been theoretically pictured'.

Further tests were then made to see whether the conditioned emotional reaction persisted, and also whether it transferred to other, similar objects, that is, whether stimulus generalization could be demonstrated. Both hypotheses were verified; the fear reaction continued, and was also shown to rabbits, fur coats, Father Christmas masks, and other furry objects. As Watson and Rayner say, 'these experiments would seem to show conclusively that directly conditioned emotional responses as well as those conditioned by transfer persist, although with a certain loss in the intensity of the reaction, for a longer period than one month. Our view is that they persist and modify personality throughout life.'

Watson and Rayner finally contrast their theory with Freud's.

The Freudians twenty years from now, unless their hypotheses change, when they come to analyse Albert's fear of the seal skin coat — assuming that he comes to analysis at that age — will probably tease from him the recital of a dream which upon their analysis will show that Albert at three years of age attempted to play with the pubic hair of the mother and was scolded violently for it. ... If the analyst has sufficiently prepared Albert to accept such a dream when found as an explanation of this avoiding tendency, and if the analyst has the authority and personality to put it over, Albert may be fully convinced that the dream was a true revealer of the factors which brought about the fear.

They conclude:

It is probable that many of the phobias in psychopathology are true conditioned emotional reactions either of the direct or of the transferred type. One may possibly have to believe that such persistence of early conditioned responses will be found only in persons who are constitutionally inferior. Our argument is meant to be constructive. Emotional disturbances in adults cannot be traced back to sex alone. They must be re-traced along at least three collateral lines — to conditioned and transferred responses set up in infancy and early youth in all three of the fundamental human emotions.

Thus Watson's theory. We may note in passing his admission of the likelihood that individual differences may play an important part in the origin of neurotic behaviour even though the phrase 'constitutionally inferior' sounds strange to modern ears and is quite unjustified. Watson was a most virulent environmentalist, attributing all of human behaviour to environmental causes; it is only in this one case that he seems to have realised the importance of individual differences. Undoubtedly he was right in this; we shall come back to this point later on.

In addition to establishing a theory of neurosis, Watson also suggested methods of curing infant, child, adolescent or adult of such neurotic fears. Unfortunately, as he says, Albert was taken from the hospital on the day that the final tests were carried out and 'hence the opportunity of building up an experimental technique by means of which we could remove the conditioned emotional response was denied us.' Watson and Rayner do however suggest some possibilities. The first suggestion relates to the methods we have already referred to as response prevention or flooding. In the article it is referred to as 'constantly confron-ting the child with those stimuli which called out the responses in the hopes that habituation would come in corresponding to "fatigue" of reflex'. A second suggestion is the method which came to be known later as desensitization; Watson and Rayner explain it as 'trying to "recondition" by feeding the subject can-dy or other food just as the animal is shown. This method calls for the food control of the subject'. In other words, we would try to condition positive reactions to the conditioned stimulus by associating it with food. This method too, like that of response prevention, has been experimented with extensively in the case of human neurotics, and has been found to work extremely well. Watson and Rayner also make other suggestions, but these are of less interest and have not been followed up in the form in which they were made.

Let us briefly summarize what Watson has attempted to do. He suggests that many if not all neurotic phobias and fears may originate through a process of Pavlovian conditioning. He suggests that through a process of stimulus generalization these fears may generalize from the original conditioned stimulus to other, similar stimuli. He suggests that these fears would last throughout life unless extinguished by some form of therapy; and he finally suggests two or more methods of treatment which should fulfil this function and which can be recommended on the basis of laboratory animal experimentation, namely the methods later to be known as response prevention or flooding and desensitization. The paper has become a classic, but it is interesting to note that Watson's theory was not accepted either by experimental psychologists or by psychiatrists and clinical psychologists. We shall look at the reasons for this rejection later on. In part it may have been due to the fact that the theory was startlingly new, and that few people, even scientists, are keen to give up their established habits of thought in favour of the new and unexplored. But in the main I think the reason for the lack of enthusiasm was the fact that there are certain difficulties in the way of accepting the theory as it stands, and that these difficulties put people off the conception of neurosis as a conditioned response. It was a pity that Watson never really came to grips with the objections, and wrote up his theory in a more extended form, taking these difficulties into account. With one exception he seems to have lost interest, and has left us little more to go on besides this short and rather inadequate paper.

The exception mentioned above is an experiment by Mary Cover Jones, a student of Watson's, who later on published her account of treatment along Watsonian lines. This is the case of Peter, a boy of two years and ten months of age, who was very much afraid of rats, rabbits and other furry animals and objects, and indeed seems to have had a pathological phobia for these stimuli. Mary Cover Jones used the two methods already suggested by Watson as well as another one which was later to become known as that of *modelling*. This method essentially uses the mechanism of imitation, the argument being that if a person who is afraid of a particular object sees other people like him in sex and age show little or no fear of the objects, then he will learn to imitate them and thus conquer his fears. This is not a technical description of the process of modelling, but it will do for the moment.

This is what Mary Cover Jones did.

> It was decided to use a rabbit for unconditioning and to proceed as follows: each day Peter and three other children were brought to the laboratory for a play period. The other children were selected carefully because of their entirely fearless attitude towards the rabbit and because of their satisfactory adjustment in general. The rabbit was always present during a part of the play period. From time to time Peter was brought in alone so that his reactions could be observed and progress noted.

It appears that this method produced improvements by more or less regular steps from almost complete terror at sight of the rabbit to a completely positive response with no signs of disturbance. Thus the method of modelling appears to have worked very well in the case of Peter.

At this point Peter was withdrawn from treatment for two months and on his return was attacked by a large dog in the presence of the nurse; both Peter and the nurse were very much frightened, and this experience seems to have reduced his recovery to the original level of extreme fear of the rabbits. This time Mary Cover Jones used the method of 'desensitization' suggested by Watson.

> Peter was seated in high chair and given food which he liked. The experimenter brought a rabbit in a wire cage as close as she could without arousing a response which would interfere with the eating. Through the presence of the pleasant stimulus (food) whenever the rabbit was shown, the fear was eliminated gradually in favour of a positive response.

This method was combined with that of modelling; 'occasionally also, other children were brought in to help with the "unconditioning".' This method worked even better; Peter developed a liking for rabbits, as was shown in some follow-up interviews.

> He showed in the last interview . . . a genuine fondness for the rabbit. What has happened to the fear of the other objects? The fear of the cotton, the fur coat, feathers, was entirely absent at our last interview. He looked at them, handled them,

and immediately turned to something which interested him more.

What would Peter do if confronted by a strange animal? At the last interview the experimenter presented a mouse and a tangled mess of angleworms.

At first sight Peter showed slight distress reactions and moved away, but before the period was over he was carrying the worms about and watching the mouse with undisturbed interest. By 'unconditioning' Peter to the rabbit, he has apparently been helped to overcome any superfluous fears, some completely, some to a less degree. His tolerance of strange animals and unfamiliar situations has apparently increased.

Here then we have an experiment apparently supporting Watson's theory very strongly. However, Mary Cover Jones indicates some element of doubt.

Peter's fear of the animals which were shown him was probably not a directly conditioned fear. It is unlikely that he ever had any experience with white rats for example. Where the fear originated and with what stimulus, is not known.

But Mary Cover Jones ends with an optimistic note:

The recent development of psychological studies of young children and the growing tendency to carry the knowledge gained in the psychological laboratories into the home and school induce us to predict a more wholesome treatment of a future generation of Peters.

Alas! although Mary Cover Jones herself was to carry on with this work and write a splendid article on 'The elimination of children's fears' in which she described several other methods of treatment, and their success, neither the conditioning theory of neurosis nor the various deconditioning and extinction methods of treatment were at all widely used until some fifty years later — recalling the well known fact that from the first discovery of the scientific principle to its every-day use usually a period of fifty years has to elapse, as in the case of the discovery of principles of electricity by Michael Faraday and the widespread use later made of electricity in everyday life as a result of the applied discoveries of Edison and others. Nevertheless, given the time distortion implicit in this general law, Mary Cover Jones was undoubtedly right and fortunately lived to see the success of her prediction, as Watson unfortunately was not able to do.

Here then we have in outline an elementary theory of neurosis as well as the adumbrations of a general theory of treatment, with quite specific suggestions as to how this treatment should proceed. The three methods mentioned, desensitization, response prevention and modelling, have in fact been the most successful weapons in our fight against neurotic disablement. In the next section we shall take up the task of bringing Watson's theory up to date, pointing out those aspects of it which have not stood the test of time and further experimentation, and enabling us to get a better understanding of the true nature of human neurosis. (Watson never in fact had any direct contacts with psychiatric patients and indeed does not seem to have done much reading in this field. Had he done so he would have realised immediately that there are many directions in which his model deviates from the kind of development which the typical neurotic disorder undergoes.) Before turning to this task, however, it may be useful to look at two case histories which illustrate rather well the way in which conditioning may work in the case of some human neurotic reactions. These two case histories are not typical, and are not meant to prove anything; they merely illustrate ways in which Watson's theory may be applicable to actual cases.

The first of the two cases in question may be called 'The case of the impotent husband.' The patient was a middle-aged man who came for treatment because he was impotent with his wife, although it soon turned out that his impotence only occurred in their home; when they went away on holiday he had no difficulty in producing a good erection. Various types of treatment were tried without success until finally, almost by accident, the truth was revealed. It appears that, several years before, the husband had been philandering and was surprised in the act by the husband of the woman in question. The husband happened to be a blacksmith of strong muscular development who proceeded to beat up the patient rather badly, producing strong fear and pain responses in the process. We may regard the act of beating up as the unconditioned stimulus, and the fear and pain reaction as the unconditioned responses in the conditioning paradigm. What was the conditioned stimulus? As it happened, the patient was looking at the wallpaper when the blacksmith began to beat him up and, as it also happened, the wallpaper in the patient's bedroom in his house had the same pattern as that of the room in which he was surprised and beaten up! We thus get the sequence of the conditioned stimulus, the wallpaper, producing feelings of anxiety in the patient, and these anxieties then making it impossible for him to achieve an erection.

The physiological mechanism through which this works is of course reasonably well understood. Sexual erection is produced via the so-called parasympathetic system, whereas fear, anxiety and so on are mediated through the sympathetic system; these two systems are largely antagonistic to each other, and the engagement of the one inactivates the other. Consequently the sight of the wallpaper would activate the sympathetic system, inactivate the parasympathetic system, and make a proper sexual response impossible. When the couple were away on holiday, there would be no such conditioned stimulus and consequently no difficulty in having intercourse. The 'treatment' consisted simply in having the room done up with a different patterned wallpaper; the patient reported no further difficulties. Obviously this is an extremely unusual case, and methods of treatment are not normally as simple as this. However it does illustrate that, occasionally at least, the Watsonian type of explanation may serve very well.

Our second case may be called 'The case of the cat woman', and refers to a severe cat phobia found in a married woman thirty-seven years old who was referred to our hospital because of a phobia for cats associated with tension, anxiety and occasional depression; it has been reported by Drs Freeman and Kendricks. This fear of cats had existed for as long as the patient could remember. 'The earliest incident she can recall is at the age of four when her father drowned a kitten in a bucket in front of her.' At the age of fourteen her parents, for some reason which is not clear, put a fur inside her bed on one occasion. 'She states that she became quite hysterical in finding it.' At the age of eighteen the patient had another fright when a cat got into her bedroom, and during her time in the WRNS (a war-time women's organisation) she was often frightened by cats, and always insisted on sleeping on the top bunk, though she did not tell anyone of her fear. These fears became worse after the age of twenty-two, and for a period of about ten years the phobia remained unchanged. However during the last year or two these fears became steadily worse.

In this last period the house next door had been empty; the grass in the gardens was very long and it became the rendez- vous for the local cats. The patient said that she was terrified by the thought that cats would spring on her and attack her. She knew that this was very unlikely in fact, but could not rid herself of the fear. At the sight of the cats she would panic and sometimes be completely overwhelmed with terror. She always walked on the roadside edge of the pavement, to avoid cats on the walls, and would never go out alone at night.

The extent of the phobia can be gauged by the fact that she would never if she could possibly help it go into any room where there was a cat. On visiting friends or relatives who had a cat, her husband or children would usually enter ahead of her to see that the cat was turned out. She was afraid to go into her garden alone, and washdays were a torment to her. She could not bear to touch any catlike fur or wear fur gloves, and felt uneasy sitting next to anyone wearing a fur coat on public transport. Pictures of cats in books or on television or the cinema made her feel uneasy. In recent months her life was filled with fear of cats, and she could think of nothing else. She interpreted any unexpected movement, shadow, or noise as due to a cat. She would be upset by her daughter's toy Koala Bear if she saw it or touched it unex- pectedly. On waking in the morning her first thought was how many cats she would meet during the day. It was as a result of this, she felt, that she would work up a fury of activity in the house and never sit still. From time to time she had terrifying night- mares, concerned with cats. This then is a typical monosymp- tomatic phobia, attached just to one object, cats, although generalising slightly to other furry things.

It is possible to regard this neurosis as having developed through a conditioning process initiated by the early traumatic event in which her father drowned a kitten in a bucket in front of her. This no doubt is the way Watson would look at this inci- dent, and possibly it played a determining part in the genesis of this particular neurosis. However there are considerable difficulties in accepting such a theory. The objections to it are manifold and it may be useful to employ this case as a kind of peg to hang our discussion of objections to Watson's conditioning theory on in the next section. We shall also later on come back to it to discuss the method of treatment which fortunately was successful and relieved the patient of her long-continued anxiety.

A new model

Of the many objections to Watson's model the first one relates to the simple fact that his 'experiment' with little Albert has been found impossible to replicate by later workers. They again did not use many cases, and it is difficult to know just what the failure was due to. It will be remembered that Watson himself said that 'We possibly have to believe that such persistence of early conditioned responses will be found only in persons who are constitutionally inferior.' Thus he may have been lucky in finding such a 'constitutionally inferior' person in little Albert, while the others, who failed to replicate his work, may have been unfortunate. There is no question at all that personality is closely related to a person's predisposition to neurotic disorders, and this must remain a likely hypothesis. The topic of personality differences, and their relation to neurosis, is so important that we shall devote a whole section of this chapter to it; consequently we will devote no more time to this particular explanation.

Another possible explanation may lie in the particular nature of the conditioned stimuli used by the psychologists who tried to replicate Watson's work. Students of phobic fears and anxieties have noted that certain objects and animals seem to feature very frequently in this context, whereas others are almost completely absent. Thus many people are afraid of spiders but hardly anyone of sheep. Many people are afraid of rats but few are afraid of common household goods, such as curtains, blocks of wood or toy ducks which were the objects used in the attempts to induce conditioned anxieties in infants made by other psychologists.

Many studies have been done to find out the major sources of phobic fears in patients. These seem to fall into quite definite groups and one statistical study has come up with the following results, as shown in Table 2. The names of the fear objects will be self-explanatory; the groups which are formed are called 'factors' and are determined by statistical analysis, not subjectively determined by the experimenter. It will be seen that the groupings

Table 2

1 *Animals*
Worms
Mice or rats
Bats
Crawling insects
Spiders
Harmless snakes
Flying insects

2 *Human hostilities*
One person bullying another
Feeling angry
Loud voice
Angry people
Losing control
Being bullied by someone
Being in a fight
Being with drunks

3 *Death and injury*
Human blood
Animal blood
Open wounds
Witnessing surgical operations
Dead animals
Receiving injections
Dead people
Medical odour
Car accidents
Suffocating

4 *Moralistic fears*
Thought of having a defective
 child
Thoughts of suicide
Sexual inadequacy (impotence
or frigidity)
Thoughts of being actually ill
Masturbation
Being punished by God

5 *Social criticism*
Feeling disapproved of
Being ignored
Being criticised
Feeling rejected by others
Looking foolish
Not being a success
Speaking before a group
Strangers

6 *Darkness*
Darkness
Being alone
Being in a strange place
Entering a room where other
 people are already seated
Going alone into a dark theatre

7 *Dangerous places*
High places
Being in an enclosed space
Being in an elevator
Crowded places
Being a passenger in an air-
 plane
Deep water

make quite good sense, and may possible be understood in terms of response generalization, that is to say the items within each group are sufficiently similar to make it quite easy to understand why a person afraid of one of these items might also tend to be afraid of the others in the same group but not of items in other groups. Thus the first factorial group seems to be defined by fears relating to small animals; the second of human relations implying hostility, disapproval, etc; the third is concerned with death and injury; the fourth with primitive, moralistic and sexual fears; the fifth with social criticism; and so on. There are one or two items which do not seem to fit in too well with this classification, but on the whole it makes remarkably good sense. It should be noted that these groupings of factors are not independent; people who have many fears in one group also tend to have fears in the others so that we emerge with a picture of people differing very much in their degree of fearfulness overall but tending to concentrate their fears more or less within one of the five groupings.

Let us now consider the second objection to Watson's theory; this is in fact related to the point just made, and forms an extension and possibly an explanation of it. Watson postulated three major original patterns of emotional reactions, namely fear, rage and love. Fear he thought was produced by simple stimuli falling into one of three categories: loud noises, loss of support, and physical constraint. All other manifestations of fear he thought were produced by conditioning, with one of the unconditioned sources being accidentally or intentionally paired with a neutral stimulus.

It is however quite unrealistic and out of line with modern research to imagine that simple sensory stimulation of this kind is the only innate source of fear reaction, or that all fear responses can be divided cleanly into innate and acquired. To take the first point first. Ethologists (investigators who study the behaviour of animals under more or less natural conditions) have provided good support for the notion of *innate fears* which may be quite specific. Thus chickens brought up from birth without any contact with other animals of their kind from whom they could in some way or other learn fear of predatory birds can be shown to react with panic flight to a cut-out resembling the shape of an eagle or a falcon being drawn along a wire over their heads. The specificity of this fear can be demonstrated by pulling the cut-out backwards, with the head following behind. In this way the silhouette does not resemble a bird plunging towards its victim, and the chicks show no fear. Natural innate fears of this kind probably exist among humans too, and it would be unrealistic to reject the possibility on *a priori* grounds.

The theory of evolution in fact would suggest that innate fears of this kind could be extremely useful in perpetuating the existence of a species, and it is interesting to note that the fears manifesting themselves as phobias in humans and listed a few pages back all would seem to have a very real and meaningful evolutionary significance. Fear of small animals like spiders or snakes may not now be reasonable, but it should be remembered that many such animals are far from harmless — scorpions, tarantulas, etc — and that in the distant past when these fears were presumably incorporated into our nervous system, many more vicious and dangerous small animals existed in the world. Fears of aggression and rejection are also very real and useful to a nomadic animal which relies a great deal on group pressures and group preservation. The same is true of the items in our fourth factor which deals with moral and sexual inadequacies which could be fatal in a primitive society. The fear of darkness and strange places, as shown in our factors six and seven, obviously has importance in indicating places where dangers might lurk. Lastly, the fear of death, wounds, blood, etc., as shown in factor three might also be interpreted with advantage as a defensive reaction. It makes good sense therefore to assume that biologically we are equipped from birth with the fear of certain animals, objects and situations which in the past have been indices of immediate danger, and which might even now fulfil a similar function, although in civilized societies these fears are probably largely obsolete.

The suggestion which emanates from these considerations is of course that many of the fears which Watson assumed to be conditioned may in fact be largely innate, although experience may exacerbate the fear-producing qualities of these stimuli. If we do have these innate fears, then the conditioning process has a much larger area to work on, besides pain, loud noises, or physical constraint. In this way it is easier to understand the large number of neurotic disorders which do not seem to involve pain in any of these forms as an unconditioned stimulus. It is true that one or

more of these supposedly 'natural' fear producers sometimes occur at the beginning of a neurosis (this is particularly true of simple phobic reactions) but it is by no means universally true of all
neuroses and is in fact probably rather unusual (except in war
neuroses). Traumatic single trial conditioning, such as we found
in the case of the erring husband who was beaten up by the
blacksmith cuckold, is relatively rare in human neurosis, yet
something like this is required by Watson's theory.

Building on this notion that some fears may be entirely or partly innate, Dr M. Seligman of the University of Philadelphia has
advanced the very appealing notion of 'preparedness'. He starts
out with pretty much the same kind of idea that we have outlined already, pointing out that in Pavlovian conditioning one conditioned stimulus is as good as another. (Pavlov wrote: 'Any
natural phenomenon chosen at will may be converted into a conditioned stimulus . . . any visual stimulus, any desired sound, any
odour and the stimulation of any part of the skin.') This does not
seem true of phobias, however:

> they comprise a relatively non-arbitrary and limited set of ob-
> jects: agoraphobia, fear of specific animals, insect phobias, fear
> of heights, and fear of the dark, etc. All these are relatively
> common phobias. And only rarely, if ever, do we have py-
> jama phobias, grass phobias, electric outlet phobias, hammer
> phobias, even though these things are likely to be associated
> with trauma in our world.

Seligman goes on to postulate that fears may not be innate, but
rather that 'phobias are highly prepared to be learned by humans,
and like other highly prepared relationships, they are selective
and resistant to extinction, learned even with degraded input,
and probably are non-cognitive.'

Some of these terms may require explanation. Conditioning in
the laboratory is usually a fairly tender plant. The time relations,
for instance, have to be just right; the conditioned stimulus must
precede the unconditioned stimulus by something like half a second or a second; if the time interval is too long or too short,
then no conditioning will take place. By suggesting that conditioning of 'prepared' reactions may take place even with
degraded inputs, Seligman means that these reactions will be
learned even although the strict rules of conditioning are not

precisely followed. It has been shown for instance that under certain circumstances such prepared reactions may be conditioned even though the interval between conditioned and unconditioned stimulus is as long as an hour. This argument gets us away from one inherent difficulty which Watson never faced, namely the problem that laboratory conditioning is a very tricky kind of thing for which very precise arrangements have to be made. In ordinary life of course one would never expect to find anything arranged in such a precise manner, and the interval between conditioned and unconditioned stimulus, for instance, may be very much longer than anything that would be tolerated in the laboratory. If we assume that 'prepared' reactions can be established by conditioning even when input is 'degraded', then we are in a much better position to generalize from the laboratory to ordinary life. By saying that phobias are non-cognitive, Seligman simply means that the fears are not rational and are not mediated by the neocortex, that is, by our normal conscious thinking apparatus.

As I have already suggested, this concept of preparedness helps to explain, among other things, why psychologists failed to get conditioning in their replication of Watson's experiment with little Albert; they used common household goods such as curtains and blocks, or a wooden duck, none of which have the 'preparedness' value of furry animals. Another problem which may be explained by this concept is the choice of conditioned stimulus: why, in a traumatic situation, does the person concerned take on one rather than another equally prominent stimulus to become *the* conditioned stimulus? On Seligman's showing, the choice would be determined very much by innate preparedness in addition to the usual chance factors. If we were frightened by a thunderstorm while out in the country, we would be more likely to pick for our conditioned stimulus a wasp flying by rather than a sheep grazing in the neighbourhood.

The notion of preparedness integrates well with the hypothesis of innate fears; presumably it is mainly a question of the degree of fear experienced which separates the two concepts. When the fear is strong upon first encountering the stimulus object, it is considered innate; when it is weak, but easily conditioned, we think of preparedness. The underlying physiological connections, and the hypothetical evolutionary development, are identical.

The concept is a valuable one, and appears necessary for a full understanding of phobic neuroses in particular. Presumably it, too, must be seen in the context of individual differences; it seems likely that personality traits are relevant to preparedness and to its role in conditioning.

One further criticism of the simple Watsonian model is the insistence on simple pain responses as providing the unconditioned response. One reason for this is probably Watson's oversimplified psychological system; another his concern with animals rather than men – except for little Albert, all his experimental work was done on rats! In the history of human neurosis, however, actual physical pain reactions are relatively rare. This is true of peace-time neuroses, at least: war neuroses often do originate in traumatic, pain-producing events, but such neuroses are known to be greatly different from the normal run of neuroses seen in hospitals. Work with animals and humans has shown that what has been called 'frustrative non-reward' has the same effects as pain, and is probably much more frequent in human affairs. This technical term means simply that we have become conditioned to expect a certain reward in a certain situation, or following certain conditioned stimuli; when this is not forthcoming our reaction is similar to that following pain. Indeed, frustrative non-reward does cause psychological pain, as anyone who has suffered it can testify. This frustrative non-reward is a much more likely candidate for providing the unconditioned part of our paradigm than is physical pain.

Conflict, too, has been shown by such eminent psychologists as N. Miller and K. Lewin to produce effects which are productive of 'psychological pain', or which are aversive and negatively reinforcing, to use more technical terminology. Particular attention has been given to what is known as 'approach-avoidance' conflict. Suppose you put a rat in a long, straight runway, with food at one end and a starting box at the other. The hungry rat soon learns to run to the food and eat it. Now provide a mild electric shock immediately in front of the food. The rat has a strong drive to approach the food but an even stronger one to avoid the shock. What will it do? Experiments have shown that this is determined by a general law which states that a spatial gradient exists, such that both approach and avoidance tendencies are stronger nearer the food than further away, but that this gradient is steeper for the avoidance than for the approach reaction.

Figure 2 illustrates this state of affairs. On the left is the starting box, on the right the goal box. It will be seen that both approach and avoidance tendencies increase in strength as they get nearer the goal, but that this gradient is steeper for the avoidance reaction. In other words, the rat gets scared more strongly as it approaches the goal box than it gets eager for the food! The relative strengths of the two tendencies determine what the rat will do. Near the starting box the approach tendency is stronger than the avoidance tendency, so it will start out running towards the goal box; gradually the difference between approach and avoidance tendency diminishes, and it will run more and more slowly, until the avoidance tendency becomes stronger (near the middle of the diagram) when the rat will begin to retreat. The rat will finally come to rest, or uneasily move to and fro, around the point where the two gradients meet. This is precisely what happens, of course; we can measure all these variables in the case of animal experiments, or even with young children, and demonstrate that this theory is along the right lines. We can even lower the avoidance gradient, e.g. by giving the rat alcohol, or some other tranquillizer; the result is shown in Figure 2 by the broken line. Now the avoidance gradient never comes up to the level of the approach gradient, and the animal reaches the goal box and eats the food. We could of course also have achieved the same end by elevating the approach gradient, for example by making the rat hungrier through starving him for twenty-four hours.

Conflict of this kind is painful (as is approach-approach conflict, in which we have a choice between two desirable objects, only one of which we are allowed to take — say two beautiful maidens only one of whom we can marry; or avoidance-avoidance conflict, in which we have to choose between two undesirable reactions, say going to prison or paying a fine!) It is important to realize that much is now known about the nature of conflict, and that the principles discovered apply just as much to human behaviour as to animal behaviour. This body of knowledge enables us to use the concept in relation to the theory of neurosis in a way that would never have been possible with the Freudian notion of conflict which has no similar fac-

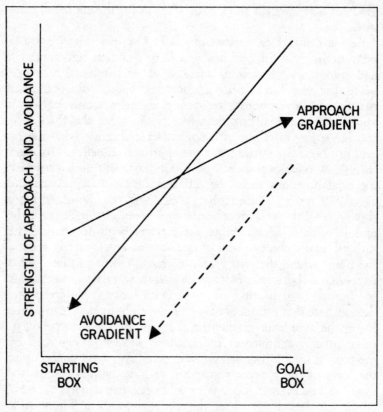

FIGURE 2
Gradients of approach and avoidance, showing
steeper slopes for avoidance. The dotted line shows
how the avoidance gradient is lowered by alcohol.

tual basis. In any case, conflict, usually of the approach-avoidance
kind, and frustrative non-reward play the part in human neurosis
which physical pain plays in animal conditioning, and sometimes
in human war neuroses; this is an important change from the simple Watsonian model.

We now come to the major objections which experimentalists
and clinicians have urged against the Watsonian theory. First let
us look at the objection made by experimentalists. It is well

known, and we have several times mentioned this fact, that *unreinforced conditioned reactions extinguish quickly*. When the conditioned stimulus is presented a number of times to the organism, without being followed by the unconditioned stimulus, extinction takes place over time, and the more frequently the pairing of conditioned stimulus and no unconditioned stimulus, the more decisive will be the weakening of the conditioned response until it is finally lost completely. This general law should be true of neurotic reactions as well but in actual fact the truth seems to be rather different.

Extinction of this kind does indeed seem to take place in neurotics, as shown by the phenomenon of spontaneous remission. This will be discussed in much greater detail later, but essentially what is meant is simply that neurotic reactions tend to die out over time even though no psychiatric treatment of any kind has been administered. Presumably this extinction occurs because the organism is frequently brought into contact with the conditioned stimulus, without any untoward consequences such as might be identified with the unconditioned stimulus and the unconditioned response. Under those conditions extinction should take place and we may thus have an explanation of spontaneous remission in this concept.

However, spontaneous remission is far from universal, and many neurotics maintain the symptoms over many years, possibly over a whole lifetime. Let us return to the example of the cat woman whose case was presented in a previous section. If we assume that the original conditioning event took place at the age of four, it is clear from the account that she encountered cats a large number of times over the years; nevertheless extinction did not take place to any degree at all. This is quite typical of most neurotic reactions. Even neurotics who try to avoid 'reality testing' cannot usually succeed in doing so completely, and will meet the feared persons, objects, or situations a number of times. On the principles of learning theory, which Watson well knew, it would be quite impossible to maintain, as he did, that 'conditioned emotional responses as well as those conditioned by transfer . . . persist and modify personality throughout life'. Quite the opposite is true; these conditioned responses should quickly extinguish and leave the individuals concerned in a pristine state of fearlessness. Failure of Watson's theory to take extinction into account is probably the major objection to it on the part of experimental psychologists.

Many attempts have been made by experimentalists to get over this difficulty and to postulate mechanisms which would not lead to extinction under these conditions. We will not deal with these attempts here because even though they might be successful they would not succeed in dealing with another problem which is even more difficult for Watson's theory. This problem is more familiar to clinicians who are in constant contact with neurotics and know something about the way the neurotic symptomatology has developed. To put it briefly, what we should expect in Watsonian terms would be a traumatic conditioning process at the beginning, followed by a gradual extinction of the feared response. What is actually found in most cases is an absence of an original traumatic conditioning situation but rather a gradual increase in fears which finally leads to a neurotic breakdown. Again the case of the cat woman may be quoted. It will be recalled that the traumatic event (if we can call it that) occurred at the age of four and that she showed fears of cats over a long period of time. These gradually increased and it was not until thirty years after the alleged traumatic event that she finally had a neurotic breakdown. In other words, what is quite typical of many neurotic disorders is a *build-up of fear over time,* with a neurotic breakdown at the end rather than at the beginning of the chain of events. It makes no difference to this account whether there is or is not a traumatic event at the beginning of the period; the important thing is the build-up of neurotic and emotional potential, increasing over time. This is quite contrary to Watson's theory or to most commonly taught learning theory, and clearly makes it impossible to accept Watson's theory as it stands. Psychiatrists clearly have good grounds for rejecting Watson's original account.

Indeed we can go one step further and point out another difficulty which is related to the first one. It is clear that a conditioned response can never be stronger than an unconditioned response. Let us consider the case of salivation following upon a bell. Originally the salivation is produced by food; salivation to the bell is a conditioned response, and it will be intuitively obvious, as well as experimentally true, that the salivation to the bell will never exceed that to the food. Similarly, in the case of little Albert, the fear of the rat should never exceed the fear produced by the unconditioned stimulus – the loud noise of the hammer banging upon the iron bar. The conditioned response derives all its strength from the original unconditioned response, and can therefore never be stronger. This is quite generally recognised in the experimental literature. What is surprising therefore is that quite frequently neurotic reactions are very much stronger than the unconditioned responses to the fear-producing stimuli which Watson's theory would hold responsible for the development of the neurosis. To take again the case of the cat woman, the reaction to the original event, the drowning of the kitten, was very much weaker than the final full blown neurosis, or even some of the intermediate stages of fear reactions to cats. This sort of thing would seem to be impossible on simple principles of conditioning and learning which Watson employed, yet it is commonplace in the development of neurotic disorders.

What we seem to observe in fact, as far as the development of neurotic reactions is concerned, is this. In many cases there is a rather slow beginning of fear reaction to certain situations, people or animals. Gradually these fear reactions become stronger and finally there may be a sudden flare-up into a proper neurotic breakdown. This contrasts vividly with the Watsonian notion of a traumatic event, building upon innate pain reactions, leading to conditioning to responses which according to theory should quickly extinguish. The contrast is a very marked one and it is small wonder that experimentalists and clinicians alike found Watson's model too simple and too unrealistic to help them much in their practical work or in their laboratory investigations.

How can we rescue the theory from this apparent impasse? I have suggested that the answer can be found in a rewriting of the law of extinction, which is in fact made necessary by a fairly large body of experimental investigations which have hitherto been rather neglected. I shall here first refer to some of the facts in question and the kind of hypothesis which they suggest; I shall then go into the reasons why the facts are as they are, and why this hypothesis can in fact be derived from higher principles. What I am suggesting is that while the presentation of a conditioned stimulus without reinforcement may lead to *extinction*, it may under certain circumstances also lead to the opposite, to an *enhancement* of the conditioned response. By this I mean that the simple presentation of the unreinforced conditioned stimulus may lead to an increment in the strength of the conditioned response, rather than to its extinction. An example may make this clear.

The experiment in question was performed by an Hungarian physiologist named S. V. Napalkov who worked with dogs and took an increase in blood pressure as his objective measure of the effects of certain conditioned and unconditioned stimuli. The unconditioned stimulus was a shot fired from a pistol (using blanks of course!) behind the ear of the dog. This stimulus produced an increase in blood pressure, but upon repetition of the stimulus habituation set in, and after 25 repetitions the dog did not respond at all to the shot; it had become completely habituated. This reaction is shown in Figure 3 under the heading 'Habituation of UCR'.

Napalkov then proceeded, on another set of dogs, to study the development of conditioned responses. In his experiments he only once paired the conditioned stimulus, which was a touch with a feather on the head of the dog, with the unconditioned stimulus, the shot fired behind the ear; after this single trial conditioning no further shots were ever fired in the whole course of the experiment. All that happened afterwards was that the conditioned stimulus, the touch of the feather, was administered a large number of times. According to orthodox learning theory extinction should have taken place very quickly, even more quickly than the habituation of the unconditioned response. However this was not so. As shown in the Figure what we get is rather the incubation or enhancement of the conditioned response; it will be seen that this response gets bigger and bigger until after 100 repetitions of the unreinforced conditioned stimulus the conditioned response is over five times as strong as it was on the original conditioning occasion. I have used the term 'incubation' to refer to this enhancement of the conditioned response under conditions when the conditioned stimulus is not reinforced; it is meant to suggest an internal development of the response independent of further applications of the unconditioned stimulus.

This experiment is mentioned only as an illustration of the kind of thing that does happen. There are many more experimental studies, some of them explicitly designed and carried out to test the hypothesis of incubation, which have given in principle

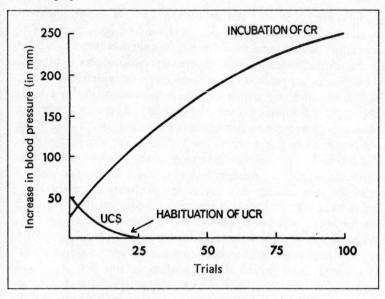

FIGURE 3
Reduction of unconditioned response through
habituation, and enhancement of conditioned
response through incubation, in dogs.

similar results, showing that under certain circumstances the administration of the unreinforced conditioned stimulus produces
enhancement rather than extinction. The facts can hardly be in
doubt any longer; we must now turn to the question of what
precisely are these circumstances which decide whether extinction or incubation takes place. Here we are on less certain
grounds, and I will simply give my own theory as to what is
happening. This theory is too new to have been properly looked
at and criticised by experimental psychologists and should
be treated with considerable caution. I believe it is along the right
lines but it will undoubtedly have to be modified in detail.

The theory I have proposed suggests essentially that we must
make a very clear distinction between conditioned responses
which act as drives, and conditioned responses which do not. Let
us go back to the dog that learned to salivate to the sound of a
bell. The bell produces salivation, but it does not produce

hunger, that is it does not produce a drive. The whole experiment only works when the dog is already hungry, that is to say working under a particular drive. The situation is quite different in the shuttlebox experiment where the conditioned stimulus (the flickering light) produces an anxiety response which itself can act as a drive, meaning that it can cause behaviour (in this case the behaviour of jumping over the hurdle). There is ample psychological literature to demonstrate that conditioned anxiety can act as a drive in this manner, and indeed anxiety and fear are the conditioned responses on which most of the work on conditioned drive has been done. Anxiety however is not the only conditioned response that can act as a drive; sex probably is another.

Let us consider a rather interesting experiment done by Dr S. Rachman in our laboratories a few years ago. He was concerned with the question of fetishism, the tendency of some patients to react with strong sexual feelings towards certain fetishistic objects (such as a shoe) which to the normal person have no sexual meaning whatsoever. Dr Rachman was interested in testing the hypothesis that fetishistic reactions are conditioned, and he arranged an experiment in which he measured the sexual reactions by using a penis plethysmograph. This is an apparatus which measures the enlargement of the penis consequent upon sexual stimulation, and records the results on a paper tape, to be read or measured later. Slides of shoes were used as the conditioned stimuli; prior to the experiment, these were shown not to have any effect on the penis whatsoever. Slides of nude women were used as unconditioned stimuli; these were found to have a very strong effect on the penis, producing marked erection. By pairing the two kinds of slides, that is, by preceding the nude women by the shoes each time, Rachman was successful in conditioning a sexual response to the slides of the shoes, and indeed he also managed to show that this reaction showed generalization, by demonstrating that sexual reactions now also followed slides of boots and other footwear.

This experiment seems to prove that conditioned sex reactions may have drive properties. It is well known that the sexual response comes in two stages: first there is *tumescence,* in the male the erection of the penis, followed by *detumescence* or orgasm. Tumescence by itself is pleasurable and sought after, as is shown by the liking for lengthy sex fore-play characteristic of males, and of their indulgence in petting and other types of non-orgasmic behaviour. In the experiment conditioned tumescence was produced, and hence it may be argued (although there is as yet no direct evidence for this) that the experiment produced a conditioned drive. The point is not an essential one for our argument and we will not pursue it here except to point out that it is noteworthy that practically all theories of neurosis nowadays implicate anxiety and sexuality as causal factors. Thus it is precisely those two responses which are likely to act as drives which are related to neurotic behaviour in modern psychiatric theorizing; this is surely significant.

How are these considerations relevant to our major problems, namely the occurrence of incubation after anxiety and other drive-producing responses? I shall here slur over some of the difficulties which arise and put the answer in a rather simplified fashion. We may go back again to the contrast between salivary conditioning and fear conditioning. In the salivary conditioning experiment, when the unconditioned stimulus (the food) is not given, then essentially nothing happens as far as the dog is concerned. There is no change in his drive level, and it may truly be said that the conditioned stimulus is not reinforced by anything.

The case is entirely different however when we turn to the shuttlebox experiment. Here the unreinforced conditioned stimulus produces a very definite and strong fear reaction which is similar to, and may be identical with, the unconditioned fear reaction produced by the shock. In other words, it would be quite wrong to say that the conditioned stimulus is unreinforced simply because the unconditioned stimulus is missing. The conditioned stimulus is being reinforced, by the unpleasant sense of fear which constitutes the conditioned response. This suggests that the reinforcement will be followed by enhancement rather than by extinction.

I have elsewhere developed this theory in some detail, including some quantitative arguments to show how this hypothesis might account for the facts as shown in Figure 2. However, this is not the place to go into details about these developments. Let the reader simply remember that conditioned fear responses (and possibly conditioned sex responses) are in an entirely different category from other types of conditioned responses, simply because they produce drive states, and that consequently the ordinary laws of extinction do not apply to these particular types of responses. Instead of extinguishing they may increase.

Along these lines we can explain both the major experimental and clinical obstacles to an acceptance of a conditioning theory of neurosis. We now see why extinction need not take place, and we also see how from a small beginning neurotic phobias and fear reactions may build up to become overwhelmingly strong, leading to a neurotic breakdown. The dogs in the Napalkov experiment shown in Figure 2 in fact did have a kind of breakdown at the end, suffering from extremely high blood pressure for a long period of time without any kind of stimulation being needed to maintain this state. This experiment incidentally also demonstrates the relevance of our theory to the so-called psychosomatic conditions about which we shall have to say something later on. Here let us simply conclude that the revamped Watsonian model does seem to give us the possibility of understanding the growth of neurotic reaction patterns, and to explain them in the terms of conditioning concepts firmly rooted in the animal and human laboratory.[1]

Many psychiatrists have criticized this whole conception as leaving out of account important cognitive variables, and as being over-simplified. We shall discuss later on whether these objections are true, and to what extent, if any, the model may have to be enlarged to include other types of variables. For the moment let us turn to a different problem, already adumbrated in this chapter, namely the nature and relevance of certain personality variables to the development of neurosis. It is impossible to understand properly the development of neurosis without hav-

[1] We might look at neurosis as the result of a kind of positive feed-back, produced by the enhancement of conditioned responses which are drive-producing. Normally the process of conditioning is productive of negative feed-back, through the extinction principle; it is when enhancement overrides extinction, under the conditions noted, that neurosis supervenes — normally only in persons whose high neuroticism predisposes them to this fate. The process in question may be made more intelligible to anyone with a schoolboy knowledge of physics by reference to Wheatstone's self-excited generator. The magnetic field in the machine is produced by an electromagnet energized by the output of the generator itself. (In more detail, an armature rotating between the poles of an electromagnet possessing some residual magnetism will generate electricity, and if the armature is connected through a commutator to the winding of the electromagnet, then the magnet is strengthened, so that more current is produced, so that the magnet is strengthened, and so on.)

ing some idea of the nature and relevance of individual differences to this general problem.

Personality and neurosis

Watson, it will be remembered, considered the possibility that little Albert's phobic fears might have been in part related to 'constitutional inferiority'. The notion that neurotics are in some sense predetermined to suffer break-down under stress is widespread. This hypothesis, in fact, lies at the basis of the widely accepted *diathesis-stress* theory of mental disorder; according to this theory people differ in predisposition (diathesis) to mental disorder, and will break down as a consequence of social stress. The greater the predisposition, the less is the stress needed to lead to breakdown. The less the predisposition, the greater the stress needed.

Figure 4 shows in diagrammatic form a model of this theory. The base line denotes the degree of genetic predisposition; against this is plotted the number of people at each level of predisposition. The large curve therefore shows how these predispositions are distributed in the population, while the small curve, cross-hatched, shows the distribution of people who are actually suffering from mental break-down. The dotted line indicates the probability of breakdown at each point of the base line, with the risk of break-down obviously increasing the further we go towards the right (the 'high predisposition' end). The factor of genetic predisposition is what we attempt to measure under the title of 'neuroticism'. High neuroticism indicates a high degree of predisposition, although stress is required in order to turn neuroticism into neurosis.

In order to put some flesh on these brief notes, we must look somewhat more closely at personality, and in particular at the influence genetic and environmental factors have on its manifestations. But before turning to this task, we must warn readers against taking Watson's term 'constitutional inferiority' too seriously. Neuroticism is indeed firmly grounded on a constitutional, genetic basis, but it would be quite wrong to consider it in terms of inferiority. To be emotionally responsive, which is the basis of 'neuroticism', is not to be inferior, and indeed in some aspects (for example, aesthetic appreciation and creation) it may stand for superiority. Biological inferiority would be in-

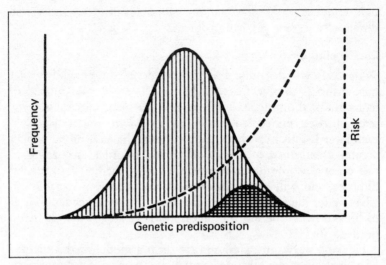

FIGURE 4
Diathesis-stress model of neurosis, indicating the
importance of genetic predisposition (diathesis)
and environmental stress.

dicated by what is called 'directional dominance' in genetics; thus
high intelligence shows directional dominance over low intelligence, and that makes sense – high intelligence obviously is
(or perhaps was!) biologically useful during the past few million
years of evolutionary selection. But low neuroticism is not direc-
tionally dominant over high neuroticism; this suggests that
biologically speaking neither end of the continuum is inferior to
the other. At some stages of development, strong fear emotions
may be more useful than a lack of fear; the one type of reaction
may lead to flight and consequent saving of one's life, the other
to disregard of danger, and death. Psychology is an objective
science and should not needlessly pass derogatory judgments on
people because of their innate behaviour patterns and reactions.

The term 'personality' is widely used by the man in the street;
does he use it in much the same way as the psychologist? In part
the answer is Yes, and in part No. The man in the street often
talks about 'strong personalities' or 'weak personalities', meaning
by that people who impress him very much, who may overawe

him, or who are very dominant, as opposed to people who are unimpressive, who are followers rather than leaders, or who are submissive. This is not the sense in which psychologists use the term. On the other hand, the man in the street would describe people in terms of traits of such as sociability, talkativeness, impulsiveness, emotionality, or courage; this is very much the kind of language the psychologist uses too. Putting it quite broadly, personality to the psychologist is closely connected with the wide field of individual differences; any form of behaviour on which people can be observed to differ falls into this field. But psychologists also tend to circumscribe the general area of individual differences somewhat by first of all ruling out differences in *ability;* these are dealt with under the concept of *intelligence.* Ideally, of course, abilities are part of personality, but the custom is to use the term only for non-intellectual differences.

Having ruled out abilities, the psychologist usually limits himself to individual differences which are socially important, or which can be shown to be related to socially important traits. People differ in the way they walk, or tie their shoe-laces, or blow their noses, but few psychologists would consider these differences worthy of study under the heading of 'personality'. If it could be shown that introverted people tended to use double ties on their shoe-laces, while extraverts did not, then one might show some interest even in such humble habits as these – not for their own sake, but because they were related to important dimensions of personality. Thus essentially the psychologist uses the term personality to refer to socially important ways in which people differ from each other in their behaviour, in their thinking, and in the manner in which they control their emotions. This is certainly not very different from at least one sort of definition the man in the street would give if he were asked to say what 'personality' meant to him.

Personality concepts are useful in describing behaviour; this is their primary function. When we say that a person is 'sociable', or has a high score on a test of the trait of sociability, we are using one word, or one score, to describe a multitude of behaviours. We mean to say that this person likes to talk to other people, that he likes going to parties, that he would be miserable alone in his room, and quite generally that contact with other people is rewarding to him. There are thousands of situations in which he could manifest his 'sociability', and knowing his degree of sociability we can predict with some accuracy how he will react. But we cannot go on to say that this concept has any causal function; it does not *explain* why a given person behaves in a sociable manner, while another one does not. Some people are tempted to say that a person likes talking to others *because* he is sociable, but this is obviously arguing in a circle – we call a person sociable because, among other things, he likes talking to people, and we cannot now turn round and say that he likes talking to people because he is sociable! This is an important limitation on the usefulness of personality concepts such as traits and types; if we want to introduce causal questions into this realm, then we need more refined analyses of the causes of behaviour.

The first attempt to solve the descriptive and causal problems of personality was made by the ancient Greeks, in their theory of types and 'humours'. Hippocrates is credited with originating the theory of the four temperaments, which was later on extended and popularized by the Greek physician Galen, who lived in the second century AD; this theory of types has given rise to terms which are still widely used, after more than two thousand years. The four temperaments are the sanguine, the melancholic, the choleric, and the phlegmatic; the descriptive meaning given to these terms by the ancient Greeks still survives in the modern usage of these terms. They tended to think of people as belonging to one or other of these types, without any possibility of mixing one with another; you could not be a bit of a choleric and a bit of a melancholic, or combine some of the traits of the sanguine person with some others of the phlegmatic. A person's type was settled at birth by virtue of certain causal influences, namely the 'humours'; these hypothetical entities bore some relation to what we would now call endocrine secretions (although the Greeks of course had only the haziest notion of what these secretions consisted of). Even so, the long life which this theory has enjoyed bears testimony to some inherent truth; with certain modifications it can still be of considerable use to modern psychology.

The main difficulty with the Greek conception, of course, lies in the fact that everybody had to fit into the four pigeon-holes provided by the theory. This clearly is not true to experience. Most of us know people who fit well into the theory – there are many cholerics, melancholics, sanguinics or phlegmatics running about, and for them the theory provides an excellent descriptive account. But equally there are even more people who do not fit into this scheme; they seem to combine features from two or even three of the types and cannot be allocated to one or the other without doing them an injustice. The answer to this problem was given by the German psychologist W. Wundt, famous for having founded the first psychological laboratory in Leipzig about a hundred years ago. He pointed out that

> the ancient differentiation into four temperaments ... arose from acute psychological observations of individual differences between people. ... The fourfold division can be justified if we agree to postulate two principles in the individual reactivity to the affects: one of these refers to the *strength*, the other to the *speed of change* of a person's feelings. Cholerics and melancholics are inclined to strong affects, while sanguinics and phlegmatics are characterized by weak ones. A high rate of change is found in sanguinics and cholerics, a slow rate in melancholics and phlegmatics.

Figure 5 shows the kind of picture Wundt describes. Where the Greeks concentrated on the four quadrants, Wundt is interested in the two dimensions or axes which run from top (emotional) to bottom (unemotional), and from right (changeable) to left (unchangeable). (Nowadays we would be more inclined to refer to extraversion and introversion as the second 'dimension' of personality, rather than to changeability and unchangeability, though it is clear that Wundt is referring to the same characteristics.) A person can be placed anywhere on these two axes, thus making the whole scheme much more flexible, and avoiding the pigeon-holing faults of the Greek scheme. Most people, in fact, would be located somewhere in the centre of the circle, not being particularly emotional or changeable, nor particularly unemotional or steadfast — just average. The trait names surrounding the circle give some indication of the nature of the four temperaments, as well as of the psychological meaning attached to the major two dimensions. This scheme has been found extremely useful in modern psychology, and with minor modifications has been shown to give an accurate account of per-

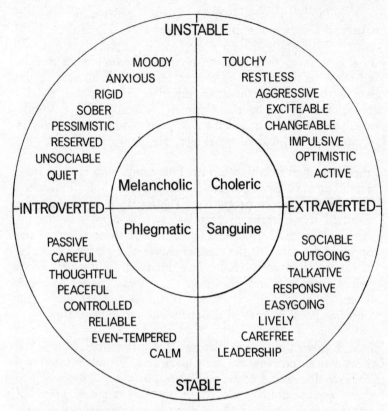

FIGURE 5
Diagram illustrating modern model of personality,
superimposed on the ancient 'four temperaments'
model.

sonality in large numbers of empirical studies of children and
adults alike.

Different psychologists have given different names to the two
dimensions. The 'emotionality' dimension is often called 'anxiety' or 'neuroticism', and the letter N will be used in referring to
it. The other dimension is now usually referred to under the title
of 'extraversion-introversion', using terms made familiar by C.
G. Jung. The letter E is often used to refer to this dimension.
These are 'type' concepts, but not in the ancient sense that

everybody must belong to one type or another; the term 'type' here simply signifies that E and N are complex combinations of trait concepts. This notion can be illustrated by referring to the way in which extraversion is based on the observed correlations between various traits such as sociability, impulsiveness, activity, liveliness and excitability. Consider Figure 6, which illustrates the hierarchical concept of personality which is now widely accepted among psychologists. At the lowest level we have specific responses, actions which an individual performs on a particular occasion. Such a response might be that while at a party he approaches and talks to a stranger. At a higher level we have the habitual response level; thus if we found that the same person frequently or habitually approached strangers and initiated a conversation we could say that this behaviour was typical of him. At a yet higher level we have the trait of sociability; this is based on the observed tendency of the same person to indulge in other sociable activities, such as having many friends, liking to go to parties and so on.

In a similar manner we can identify and measure other trait concepts, such as those indicated in Figure 5. It is now a matter of empirical observation whether or not these traits are themselves correlated; in other words, is it true that a person who is sociable also tends to be impulsive, physically active, lively, excitable? We do in fact find that such relations exist, and in order to explain them we use the concept of the extraverted type. It will be seen that this theory is based on empirical observation throughout, followed by statistical analysis of the observed relations; there is nothing airy-fairy or speculative about it. We are dealing with hard facts, observations of the behaviour patterns of many thousands of individuals, belonging to many different cultures. Indeed, similar behaviour patterns have even been observed in monkeys, so that we may assume that there is some strong biological causation behind our observed patterns.

There are many ways of measuring such personality traits and types as those mentioned. Observation and rating of actual behaviour is one such method; it is quite complex and difficult, and very time-consuming, but of course possesses obvious advantages. Under certain circumstances personality questionnaires may be used; it is of course possible to fake one's answers, and when questionnaires are used for the purposes of occupational

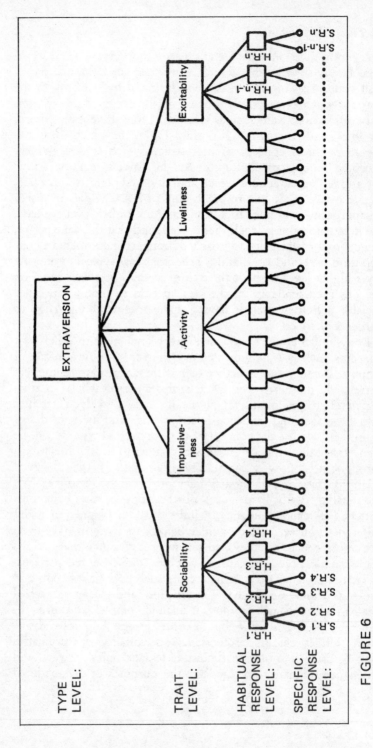

FIGURE 6
A hierarchical model of personality showing extraversion as a combination of several different traits.

selection faking does in fact often take place. But when questionnaires are used for experimental purposes, the great majority of people tend to give truthful answers, and questionnaire measurement can be extremely useful under these circumstances. It is possible to compare the results of these two types of investigation; for instance, we can ask a group of people to nominate extreme extraverts and extreme introverts among their friends, and then administer questionnaires to the people chosen. It is generally found that those nominated as extraverts have high extraversion scores on the questionnaire, while those nominated as introverts have high introversion scores. There are many other ways of demonstrating the accuracy of questionnaire results, and these have on the whole shown that questionnaires, when properly constructed and administered, can give a very accurate picture of a person's personality.

Below is given a very short questionnaire for the measurement of E and N; the first six questions relate to N, the next six to E. Every 'Yes' answer counts one point for the relevant type. A score of 2, 3 or 4 would suggest that the person achieving such a score was ambivert, i.e. middling in his standing on E or N. Scores of 0 or 1 suggest a stable person (on N), or an introverted one (on E). Scores of 5 to 6 suggest an emotional person (on N), or an extraverted one (on E). The questionnaire is given merely to illustrate the kinds of questions asked; it is much too short to make self-diagnosis possible.

Questionnaire

1　Do you sometimes feel happy, sometimes depressed, without any apparent reason?　　Yes　No

2　Do you have frequent ups and downs in mood, either with or without apparent cause?　Yes　No

3　Are you inclined to be moody?　　Yes　No

4　Does your mind often wander while you are trying to concentrate?　　Yes　No

5　Are you frequently 'lost in thought' even when supposed to be taking part in a conversation?　　Yes　No

6   Are you sometimes bubbling over with
    energy and sometimes very sluggish?   Yes   No

7   Do you prefer action to planning for action?   Yes   No

8   Are you happiest when you get involved in
    some project that calls for rapid action?   Yes   No

9   Do you usually take the initiative in making
    new friends?   Yes   No

10 Are you inclined to be quick and sure in
    your actions?   Yes   No

11 Would you rate yourself as a lively
    individual?   Yes   No

12 Would you be very unhappy if you were
    prevented from making numerous social
    contacts?   Yes   No

Are these typologies of any social relevance? A few examples must suffice to answer this question in the affirmative. Let us look at two very large groups in society which cause a great deal of trouble and expense — neurotics and criminals. It has been found that a high proportion of neurotics come from the 'melancholic' quadrant, that is, they tend to be emotional, introverted people. On the other hand, a high proportion of criminals come from the 'choleric' quadrant, made up of emotional, extraverted people. Follow-up studies have shown that these relations can be shown to hold even when the personality diagnosis is made at a very early age, say at the age of ten. These children who are rated emotional and introverted tend to become neurotics when adult, while those who are rated emotional and extraverted have a more than average chance of becoming criminals when adult. Thus there is a close connection between personality and such socially important categories as neurosis and crime.

In the field of employment and job selection there are also important connections with personality. One investigator decided to follow up Jung's suggestion that artists tend to be emotional and introverted. Hundreds of students in a large university department concentrating on the visual arts (primarily painting) were rated for originality and excellence of work by their teachers; the 15 students with the highest marks were all concentrated in the 'melancholic' quadrant, in other words they were both emotional and introverted. In another study paratroopers and commandos were investigated; they tended to fall almost without fail into the phlegmatic quadrant, among the stable extraverts. High-ranking business executives were found to be predominantly stable introverts. Examples could be multiplied to show that personality is a very important concept in relation to a person's work and social behaviour.

To what extent is our personality determined by genetic causes, and to what extent by environmental ones? In so far as personality differences are caused by innate factors, so far does personality appear to be immutable. When environmental factors assume prominence, the picture changes; clearly behaviour patterns which have been produced by environmental factors can be eliminated by environmental factors of a different kind. If you are unsociable because of the social environment in which you grew up, a change of environment may change you into a more sociable person. If you are timid and withdrawn because you were bullied at school, you may change these behaviour patterns when you leave school and move among more accommodating people. It may of course be possible that patterns of behaviour acquired early are more difficult to change later on, once you have formed these habits of conduct, but in principle there seems to be no good reason why extensive changes should not be possible.

What, then, is the evidence regarding heredity, and its influence on personality? The best evidence here comes from studies of twins. Nature has performed an exciting experiment for us by providing two kinds of twins – identical or monozygotic (MZ) and fraternal or dizygotic (DZ). Identical twins are always of the same sex, and are practically identical as far as heredity is concerned. They originate from a single ovum, fertilized by a single sperm; the fertilized ovum then splits up into two (or occasionally more) separate individuals. Fraternal twins may be of the same sex, but they may also be of different sex; on the average, they share heredity only to the extent of 50%, no more than ordinary brothers and sisters not born at the same time. Fraternal twins originate from two separate ova, fertilized by two separate sperms.

These accidental experiments of nature enable us to study the influence of heredity along two rather different routes. We can study identical twins who have been separated at birth or shortly after, and who have been brought up in quite different environments by foster parents or in orphanages or in some other way. Under these conditions, any similarities between them could only be the effect of heredity, not environment, seeing that they did not share a common environment (except of course while within the womb).

The other method of study makes use of comparisons between identical twins, on the one hand, and fraternal twins, on the other. Let us suppose that a given trait, say sociability, is due entirely to environmental causes. Now the only difference between identical and fraternal twins is of course that the former share more heredity in common; this is irrelevant to our hypothetical trait, and consequently identical twins would be no more alike with respect to sociability than would fraternal twins. But let us now suppose that heredity plays an important part in producing differences in sociability between people; in that case we would expect identical twins to be much more alike than fraternal twins, simply because they share more common heredity. The general rule might be stated as follows: the greater the similarity between identical twins, as compared with fraternal twins, the greater the influence of heredity. This relation can be expressed numerically, and may be used to estimate the relative contribution of nature and nurture, heredity and environment.

Such formulae make certain assumptions, but these can of course be checked. For instance, they assume that there is no 'assortative mating', and that men and women marry in a random manner as far as personality traits are concerned. (There is no particular reason why introverted men should marry introverted women, or extraverted ones, for that matter.) Is this assumption true? When personality questionnaires are given to large samples of married people, and personality scores correlated, it is found that there is indeed no correlation at all for extraversion-introversion; mating is quite random as far as this major dimension of personality is concerned. The position is slightly different for neuroticism (emotionality *v.* stability); here there is some evidence for assortative mating, the more emotional tending to marry the more emotional, and the more stable tending to marry the more stable. But this tendency is very weak, and can easily be accommodated in the formula. Altogether, assortative mating is curiously weak or absent in our society; most people would probably have expected either a tendency for like to marry like, or else the opposite. Like does marry like with respect to intelligence, where quite high correlations are found between spouses, but not with respect to personality.

What is the outcome of the many studies which have been carried out in this country and in the United States, where most of the work has been done? (There have also been a few studies on the European continent.) Let us take first the experiments using identical twins brought up in separation. Here the outcome is rather curious; it has been found that twins brought up in separation are if anything slightly more alike than are twins brought up together! Both groups, in fact, are very similar with respect to extraversion and neuroticism; knowing one twin, you could give a very good guess about the personality of the other. How is it possible that environment not only fails to make twins growing up together more alike, but may actually make them somewhat more different than twins growing up in separation? The answer may lie precisely in the great similarity that exists between twins; often identical twins resent the fact that they are not regarded as separate persons, and tend to stress any small and accidental differences in behaviour that may occur simply in order to appear different. Thus one twin may take over the negotiations with the outer world, while the other takes over the internal management of the affairs of the twins. This parcelling out of roles is often facilitated by the fact that identical twins interfere with each other in the womb more than do fraternal twins, due to the fact that they share a common placenta in most cases; thus one twin may deprive the other of part of the blood supply, leading to differences in birth weight which are often correlated with intelligence, dominance and so on. Thus, contrary to expectation, identical twins may share an environment in the womb which makes for *greater* differences than that shared by fraternal twins. The slight differences caused in this way may then lead the twins to emphasize and exaggerate these differences. Whatever may be the truth about these complex matters, there is no doubt that the evidence from identical twins brought up in separation demonstrates very clearly that heredity plays a very important part in producing differences in personality between people.

Experiments comparing identical and fraternal twins bear out this conclusion. Out of some twenty studies, there is not one in which the correlations for identical twins have not been larger, and usually much larger, than those for fraternal twins. This is true not only for the major personality variables, such as extraversion-introversion and neuroticism-stability; it applies equally to a large number of different traits that have been measured in various ways. The only personality measures which have on the whole failed to show much in the way of a difference between identical and fraternal twins have been projective tests, such as the Rorschach and the TAT, and expressive tests, such as graphology. But here the reason would seem to be not so much that there are no differences between the different kinds of twins, but rather that these tests possess low reliability and little validity; in other words, they fail to measure personality with any precision, and consequently cannot be used to prove anything regarding the importance of heredity or environment.

When proper personality tests are used, whether questionnaires or objective experimental testing procedures, results always support the proposition that heredity plays a most important part in producing differences in personality between people. It is not easy to give a numerical value to the proportional importance of nature and nurture; results depend in part on the actual instruments used for carrying out the measurement, and the numbers of twin pairs have often been too small to give very accurate results. The minimum value for the contribution of heredity is something like 50 per cent, with the maximum in the region of 80 per cent. Probably something like 65 per cent would be the best guess which one can make at the moment; this would apply to extraversion-introversion and neuroticism-stability. Simpler traits, like sociability or impulsiveness, give lower values, but still up to the 50 per cent mark. Thus there can be no doubt that personality has a hard core of innately determined behaviour patterns. This hard core (the genotype, as geneticists call it) interacts with the environment to produce the actually observed behaviour (the phenotype).

These findings raise some interesting problems. It is of course quite impossible to inherit conduct; we can only inherit physical structures that can be identified by the physiologist or the

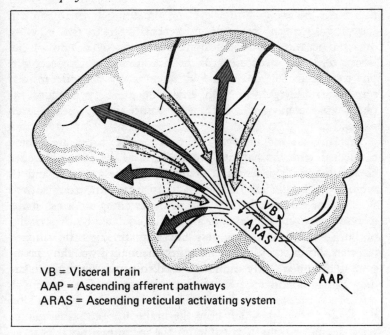

VB = Visceral brain
AAP = Ascending afferent pathways
ARAS = Ascending reticular activating system

FIGURE 7
The physiological basis of extraversion and neuroticism.

anatomist. Yet what we measure when we talk about personality
is conduct, or behaviour; this suggests that there must be some
physical structures in our nervous system which mediate
behaviour of the kind which causes us to diagnose a person as extraverted or introverted, neurotic or stable. We now have some
idea which are the structures involved. Consider Figure 7, which
is a picture (in very diagrammatic form) of the cortex and the
spinal cord. At the base of the brain, note the so-called visceral
brain or limbic system. This co-ordinates the activities of the
autonomic system, which governs the expression of the emotions,
through its two parts, the sympathetic and the parasympathetic
systems. Emotions such as fear and anger are always accompanied
by such physical manifestations as increased heart beat, more
rapid breathing, sweating, the cessation of digestion, dilation of
the pupil, etc.; these are produced by the sympathetic system, and
coordinated by the visceral brain. The parasympathetic calms

things down, brings heart beat and breathing back to normal, starts the digestion up again, and generally relaxes the organism once the occasion for the emotional outburst is over. This visceral brain, and the structures of the autonomic system, are the physical basis for individual differences in neuroticism and stability; in interaction with environment, they produce the phenotypic behaviour which we measure with our questionnaires.

Extraversion and introversion, on the other hand, are closely connected with the habitual arousal level of the cortex. We are all familiar with different arousal levels – we are tense and all wound up, highly aroused, prior to an important examination; we are relaxed and drowsy late in the evening in front of the television screen. The level of arousal is regulated by the activity of the so-called ascending reticular activating system, situated close to the visceral brain. Incoming messages from the various parts of the body, the eyes, ears, etc., go directly to the brain, but they also send collaterals to the reticular system. This system in turn sends messages to the cortex (symbolized in Figure 7 by the shaded arrows) which keep the brain in a receptive state of arousal, thus making it possible for the incoming messages to be received and acted upon. The higher the arousal level, the better is the brain able to function.

Introverts have higher habitual levels of arousal; hence they tend to be better at learning, conditioning and remembering. The cortex also has the function of keeping the lower levels in check; hence the behaviour of introverts is more inhibited than that of extraverts. An illustration may make clearer what goes on. Alcohol makes people more extraverted, while the amphetamines, which are stimulant drugs, have the opposite effect; they increase the level of cortical arousal, and make people more introverted. So does nicotine, and caffeine; hence students trying to study hard for an examination tend to smoke and drink coffee to keep awake, and to learn better. Here we have one answer to our question of whether personality can change; by giving people depressant or stimulant drugs we can alter the physical basis of their personality, and thus alter their behaviour. Another method, slightly gruesome, is that of brain operation. Lobotomy or leucotomy operations are sometimes carried out on patients suffering from severely inhibited behaviour; in this operation the pre-frontal areas of the brain are cut off from the rest, thus reducing the amount of cortical arousal, and making people more extraverted.

But of course we do not have to go to such extreme lengths to produce changes in behaviour and personality. Even though heredity plays an enormously important part in producing differences in personality, environment, too, is important. Thus we would expect important changes to take place with age; the older a person is, the longer will environment have had opportunities to make him change in socially approved and personally rewarding ways. By and large this is true; as people get older, they get less emotional and neurotic, and less extraverted. Adolescence, the time of *Sturm und Drang*, shows the highest levels of neuroticism and extraversion; gradually people simmer down and present a less explosive mixture. No wonder that it is in adolescence that most crimes are committed. Indeed, most antisocial behaviours are found in young people; as they get older they learn (or are conditioned) to make their peace with society.

How does this picture of personality relate to our theory of neurosis? The connection is very clear. We picture neurotic reactions as conditioned emotional responses; clearly the two major personality patterns, neuroticism and introversion, are closely related to these two types of reactions. Persons high on neuroticism are characterized above everything else by strong, long-lasting emotions; these are typical reactions in painful, fear-producing, conflictful situations which constitute the 'stress' in our diathesis-stress model. Such persons are obviously more likely to form strong and long-lasting conditioned emotional responses under these conditions; they are *predisposed* to become neurotic in ways that the low N scorer, with his inadequate emotional response to similar situations, is not. Equally, introverts, because of their high level of cortical arousal, form conditioned responses more quickly and more strongly, and extinguish them less readily than do extraverts; this inevitably makes them more likely to form those conditioned emotional responses which in our theory constitute the neurotic disorder. There is now much evidence to verify the assumption that introversion and conditioning are firmly related, and there is no doubt that the great majority of neurotics are in fact introverted and high on neuroticism when tested. As already noted, it has also been found that when schoolboys are assessed for these two personality traits at the age of ten and then followed up, those who turn out to become neurotics within the next thirty years or so tend to come overwhelmingly from the high N/low E group; that is to say, it is this group that is predestined genetically to make up the majority of our future neurotics. Some are saved by not being exposed to strong stress and some of those who are not in the high N/low E quadrant do become neurotic through being exposed to particularly strong stresses; but on the whole the predictive accuracy is surprisingly high.

At the moment we are concerned mainly with the 'melancholic' quadrant, the high-N introverts who are likely to break down, showing the typical major patterns of neurosis – anxiety state, obsessive-compulsive disorder, reactive depression, phobias, and so forth. This range of disorders will be referred to as 'dysthymia', disorders of mood or emotion. Some major neurotic disorders, however, tend to fall into the high-N group of extraverts, for example hysteria, psychopathy, personality disorder, and above all criminality. This group will be dealt with in a separate chapter, and it will be noted that people of this kind require rather different types of treatment, as compared with dysthymics. Our next chapter will outline some of the more widely used methods of behaviour therapy which have been found useful in the treatment of dysthymic disorders.

4 Methods of Behaviour Therapy

Desensitization

We have so far considered the general theory which tells us how neurotic symptoms are produced; we must now discuss in detail the available methods for extinguishing these so-called symptoms. The term 'symptom' is in fact a misnomer, if our theory is correct; these 'symptoms' are not symptomatic of anything else but do in fact constitute the disorder. When Freud developed his theory he followed the medical practice of distinguishing between symptoms and underlying causes; in his theory the anxiety and the other observable behaviours which make up the neurosis were merely symptomatic of some underlying disease process, just as a fever is merely a symptom of some disease or other. Just as the physician does not treat the fever but the underlying disease, so Freud thought we should treat whatever underlies the neurotic symptoms. Symptomatic treatment, he was convinced, leads nowhere; the symptom might be suppressed, but either it would return after a while (relapse) or another symptom would take its place (symptom substitution).

In his theory the underlying 'disease' was made up of unconscious complexes, such as the famous Oedipus complex, the desire on the part of the male child to possess his mother sexually and to murder his father. Because of the obviously greater physical power of the father, this wish is repressed into the unconscious, but remains active, and later on may be reawakened and give rise to the symptoms which are observable. If this theory were correct, then it would follow that only by dealing with this underlying complex (or the other complexes in which Freud believed, such as the Electra complex in women) could we effect a permanent cure.

During the days of psychoanalytic supremacy in the psychiatric world, it was indeed confidently claimed that cures of neurotic disorders (and even of psychotic disorders) could be accomplished by the psychoanalytic method of making such complexes conscious and reintegrating them emotionally with the conscious life of the patient. This hope, alas, was unfulfilled; empirical studies of the actual effectiveness of psychoanalytic and other psychotherapeutic methods have failed to show any improvement in patients treated by psychoanalysis which could not also be found in patients receiving no psychiatric treatment at all (spontaneous remission). We shall look at some of the details of this type of research later on; here let us merely note that in recent years psychoanalysts have become much more modest in their claims, and now merely assert that their methods make the patient a 'better person' (leaving it open what is meant by being a better person), though they can do very little about the actual symptoms of which he complains. The assumption is still made that the symptoms are in fact 'symptoms', that is that there is some underlying disease process identified with Freudian complexes.

It is this hypothesis which is contradicted by the theory underlying the methods of behaviour therapy. The anxieties, the reactive depression, the obsessive-compulsive behaviour, and all the other neurotic emotions and behaviours of the patients are held, according to this theory, to be nothing more than conditioned emotional responses, or their reactions to such conditioned emotional responses, bearing in mind of course the additional complications introduced by such factors as preparedness, incubation of anxiety and so on. If this is so, then the symptoms are indeed the disease, and are not 'symptomatic' of anything. A cure, according to this theory, is effective once the symptoms have been removed. We shall continue to use the term 'symptom' because of its usefulness, and because it has received universal acceptance. Nevertheless the reader will bear in mind that these so-called symptoms are not symptomatic of anything except themselves.

There are ten major ways in which behaviour therapy differs from psychotherapy. The first of these differences relates to theory. Psychotherapy is based on an inconsistent theory never properly formulated in postulate form, and never given a proper empirical test. Behaviour therapy is based on a consistent, properly formulated theory leading to testable deductions. Put in another way, behaviour therapy follows the usual dictates of scientific method while psychotherapy does not.

Secondly, psychotherapy is derived from clinical observations made without the necessary control observations or experiments. Freud generalized to all human nature from his observations on a small number of neurotic upper-middle-class Viennese men and women; he never worried about extrapolating from this very small data base to the whole of the human race. The principles of behaviour therapy are derived from experimental studies specifically designed to test basic theories and the deductions made therefrom. Here again, therefore, behaviour therapy obeys the dictates of scientific method whereas psychotherapy does not.

The third major difference we have already discussed. Psychotherapy considers symptoms a visible upshot of unconscious causes ('complexes'). Behaviour therapy considers 'symptoms' as unadaptive conditioned responses. Related to this is the fourth major difference. Psychotherapy regards symptoms as evidence of *repression*, whereas behaviour therapy regards symptoms as evidence of faulty learning or conditioning.

The fifth difference relates to symptomatology. Freud and most psychotherapists believe that symptomatology is determined by defence mechanisms, that is by the various ways in which the mind defends itself against the repressed, unconscious material trying to get into consciousness. Behaviour therapists believe that symptomatology is determined by individual differences in the ease of difficulty with which a person acquires conditioned responses, and the degree of responsiveness of his autonomic system, as well as accidental environmental circumstances. It follows, as the sixth major difference, that to the psychotherapist all treatment of neurotic disorders much be *historically* based, whereas for the behaviour therapist all treatment of neurotic disorders is concerned with habits existing at *present*; the historical development is largely irrelevant for treatment, although it may be of interest theoretically.

To the psychotherapist, it appears that cures are achieved by handling the underlying (unconscious) dynamics, not by treating the symptom itself. For the behaviour therapist, cures are achieved by treating the symptom itself directly, by extinguishing unadaptive conditioned responses, and establishing desirable conditioned responses. It follows, eighthly, that for the psychotherapist interpretation of symptoms, dreams, acts, etc. is an important element of treatment, whereas to the behaviour therapist interpretation, even if not completely subjective and erroneous, is irrelevant.

Two further beliefs characterize the psychotherapist. The first is that symptomatic treatment leads either to relapse or to the appearance of new symptoms (symptom substitution). He also believes that transferences are essential for cures of neurotic disorders; that is to say, he considers that the personal relations established between therapist and patient are vital in reviving the unconscious memories through transference of the accompanying emotions to the therapist. Behaviour therapists believe that symptomatic treatment leads to permanent recovery provided autonomic as well as muscular (motor) maladaptive conditioned responses are extinguished, and he considers that personal relations are not essential for cures of neurotic disorders, although they may be useful in certain circumstances. These are the ten major differences between psychotherapy and behaviour therapy. To these we might add one further point which we shall elaborate later on. It is simply that by and large psychotherapy does not work very well, whereas behaviour therapy does. In addition to amplifying this point, we shall also later on discuss some of the possible objections that psychotherapists may raise against symptomatic treatment, and also some ethical questions that arise. However in this chapter we shall be concerned more with the presentation of the actual methods of behaviour therapy (or at least some of these methods; learning theory has been prolific in suggesting methods of treatment, and not all of those which have proved fruitful can be discussed in the scope of a small and popular book such as this).

The most widely used of all the methods of behaviour therapy is undoubtedly that of *desensitization*. We have already come across it in connection with the suggestions made by Watson and Rayner about possible treatments of little Albert's rat phobia, and have seen the method to work in Mary Cover Jones's treatment of Peter and his rabbit phobia. The method was rediscovered and adapted to clinical work by Dr (later Professor) Joseph Wolpe, a South African psychiatrist who later on came to England and is now teaching at Temple University in Philadelphia, USA. He had been trained as a psychoanalyst but, like many others, found the treatment ineffective, lengthy and expensive. Looking for alternatives, he carried out some experimental work with cats, following up Masserman's work which we have already mentioned. This, and the consideration of learning theory principles led him to the elaboration of his methods which were published in 1958 in book form under the title *Psychotherapy by Reciprocal Inhibition*. Simultaneously but independently, similar work was being carried out by my colleagues in the Psychology Department of the Maudsley Hospital and the London University Institute of Psychiatry, the two of which are closely related in location and spirit. Our work was influenced not only by Watson and Mary Cover Jones, but also by Alexander Herzberg, a German refugee psychiatrist who settled in England and used what he called a method of 'active' psychotherapy.

In this, patients with specific fears and anxieties were given graduated tasks, starting with relatively easy tasks producing little anxiety, and working up to more and more difficult ones. Thus a patient showing a fear of open spaces would be instructed to set foot outside his door and take two or three steps in either direction and then go back. If he found this too stressful, he might be accompanied by his wife or friend. Gradually the range would be extended to five or six steps, then to ten, then to twenty, then to going to the end of the street, then going round the square. Gradually the patient would work up towards complete freedom of fear under these circumstances. The therapist would of course always be ready with reassurance and advice, but these graduated tasks were a most important part of the treatment process. As we shall see, Wolpe arrived at a similar concept of gradual working up from low anxiety to high anxiety behaviour, accompanied by relaxation exercises, although he emphasised practising these behaviours in imagination, whereas Herzberg and our early work preferred *in vivo* exercises – actual practising of the behaviours to be learnt.

Wolpe's animal experiments essentially consisted in showing that Masserman's hypothesis of conflict was not necessary to explain his results. He fed cats in a certain room in his laboratory, then gave them shocks preceded by a conditioned stimulus. He found that the shock produced strong conditioned avoidance reactions not only to the conditioned stimulus, which was a tone, but also to the whole situation, the room and the experimenter. He found it quite unnecessary to produce the kind of conflict which Masserman had produced, between eating and receiving a noxious stimulus at the same time: animals so treated did not behave any differently. Wolpe then attempted to cure the very strong avoidance and anxiety reactions produced by the conditioning process by feeding the animals in the presence of relatively weak anxiety responses. He started at some distance from the room where the conditioning had taken place, then gradually brought them nearer and nearer, taking care to feed them each time and stroking them and in other ways 'reassuring' them. In this way he managed gradually to coax them back into the laboratory, and removed their conditioned fear responses completely.

This work (which is here described only very cursorily) led him to enunciate the following general principle: 'If the response antagonistic to anxiety can be made to occur in the presence of anxiety-evoking stimuli so that it is accompanied by a complete or partial suppression of the anxiety responses, the bond between these stimuli and the anxiety responses will be weakened.' This is the principle of desensitization or 'reciprocal inhibition' as Wolpe calls it. In other words, we have conditioned an avoidance response and an unpleasant emotional reaction to a previously neutral stimulus, namely the conditioned stimulus; this anxiety and avoidance reaction is now our 'neurosis'. We get rid of it by a process of counter-conditioning, by attempting to condition pleasant and positive reactions to the same stimulus. These positive and pleasant reactions will lessen the force of the negative and unpleasant reactions previously conditioned, and the longer we continue, the greater will be the extinction of these negative and unpleasant reactions. In the case of the cats, feeding them at some distance from the laboratory produces a slight degree of anxiety (because of the nearness of the conditioned stimulus) but the pleasant reactions produced by the feeding overshadow the slight anxiety and therefore produce a positive conditioned feeling towards the laboratory. In this way we can now bring the cats nearer and nearer to the room where the original conditioning took place, until finally the whole of the unpleasant conditioned reaction has been suppressed or extinguished. The similarity to Herzberg's method will be apparent.

For humans, Wolpe makes two suggestions. In the first place, the therapist constructs a hierarchy of anxiety-producing situations or stimuli, ranging from the lowest to the highest. He then works through these systematically, starting at the bottom, and working up towards the top, never proceeding so hurriedly that the patient experiences intolerable anxiety. If that should happen, the whole course of the treatment would be endangered. The other suggestion made by Wolpe is that the patient should be trained in relaxation, in lessening the tenseness of the muscles of his body which usually accompanies unpleasant emotions and anxiety. Relaxation is thus opposed to anxiety, and we attempt to condition muscular relaxation to those stimuli which at the beginning produce anxiety in the patient. This combination of hierarchies and relaxation constitutes in essence the method which Wolpe introduced into psychiatry.

An example will make it clearer just what happens in an actual case. Let us return to the case of the cat woman whom we left in an earlier chapter at the age of thirty-two, mortally afraid of cats and having suffered from this phobia on and off for almost thirty years. Her plan of treatment was elaborated on the following basis. It was considered that the weakest point of the 'stimulus gradient' (that is, the anxiety hierarchy) would be material that had some of the texture of fur without looking like it – for example, velvet. A series of pieces of material was prepared, graded in texture and appearance from something most unlike cat fur to something very like it. The patient would then be instructed to handle the material in order of similarity to cat fur, and before she proceeded with the next piece in the series would have to be quite sure that she felt no uneasiness whatsoever in handling it. After overcoming the fear reactions to handling catlike fur, she would be presented with a toy kitten, and with pictures of cats, until they caused no anxiety. When this state was achieved she would be shown a live kitten, and gradually taught to approach and touch it. Having accomplished this she would be asked to take it home and keep it. As it grew, so the generalization to large cats would occur and finally she would be free from her phobia for cats.

This plan was followed with results as discussed below by Drs Freeman and Kendrick, who carried out the treatment.

At his interview with the patient the psychologist outlined the programme he had formulated and gave the eventual aim as being that she should be able to touch a fully grown cat without distress. The patient felt that the method seemed reasonable to her, but was very sceptical about the outcome; she could not conceive of herself as ever being able to touch even a kitten.

The psychiatrist then began the presentation of stimuli at the Day Hospital, and told the patient to handle each material in turn, until it caused her no uneasiness. When a glove made of rabbit fur was eventually offered the patient was so upset by it that she wrapped it up in newspaper. However, another patient encouraged her by putting the glove on himself and persuading her to stroke it. Within a few days it had ceased to cause her any unpleasant feelings.

The patient's intelligent cooperation in the procedure was illustrated by her experience with pictures of cats. When this point was reached she was advised to obtain some large pictures and put them up at home. She was a little overenthusiastic, and arranged nine in different parts of the house, particularly in corners where they would surprise her. This proved rather distressing for her and she had to take down some of the more frightening ones, but in the course of the next week or so she became used to all of them.

At the end of three weeks, fur, toys, and pictures had all been fully assimilated and a significant lessening in anxiety had already occurred. She was much less preoccupied with cats in general and her family had noticed that she was altogether more cheerful. She could walk within about 10 yards of a cat without flinching, and when opening the curtains in the mornings her first reaction was no longer to look around the garden for cats.

The rapidity of response so far seemed remarkable, and the patient now felt ready to deal with a live kitten. One of a suitably placid disposition was obtained and the patient was brought into the room, where she saw it resting on the lap of one of the nurses. She sat down next to the nurse, stroked the kitten herself, and then took it on her own lap. During this process she became very emotional, both laughing and crying, but this passed off in a few minutes, and she explained afterwards that it was not from distress, but from relief at having done something of which she imagined herself incapable. She later described this as 'one of the greatest days of my life'.

In the next two days she looked after the kitten at the Day Hospital and then took it home, where it has remained since. This occurred one month after her first attendance, and during the next two months she continued to attend twice weekly, but mainly for the art classes, in which she was very interested. During this time she was assessed weekly by the psychiatrist, and her improvement was seen to be continuing. She said that she felt as though a cloud had been lifted from her, and she had stopped biting her nails for the first time in her life.

One month after taking the kitten home she had her second interview with the psychologist. She stated that she no longer walked along the edge of the pavement, and could wear fur gloves and sit next to people in fur coats without feeling uneasy. She was no longer upset by pictures or films of cats and could consider some of them as beautiful creatures. She could pass near to a full-grown cat without panicking, and felt she would be able to go out alone at night, but her family had not let her try so far. She had stopped having cat nightmares; however, she dreamed without distress of kittens and later of full-grown cats.

On two successive nights the following week she had aggressive dreams concerned with her father and was very miserable in the intervening day. In one dream she was murdering her father with a poker. In recounting these she stated that she had often had feelings of this sort when her father was alive, but had not allowed herself to express any hostility against him.

Ten weeks after beginning treatment she touched a full-grown cat for the first time. She was so thrilled by this that she felt like running down the street and telling everyone and then was reluctant to wash her hands afterwards. She then touched her mother's black cat, though cats of this colour had been the ones which previously frightened her most. Whereas previously all cats had an almost uniformly sinister aspect, she could now see individual differences.

After three months she discontinued attendance at the Day Hospital, but came to report progress to the psychiatrist at intervals of three weeks, lengthening to one month. She states that her life has been completely transformed, and that she no longer goes round in a state of fear. Nor does she feel the need any longer to occupy herself in constant activity inside the house to relieve her anxiety. The kitten has grown considerably, and she has no difficulty in dealing with it. At the end of the fifth month from beginning treatment she has been out by herself at night, even in dimly lit streets. The only episode which caused her any distress was going into the back garden at night on her own. At the end of the eighth month (and two months after the previous interview) she remained well, except for a brief relapse, which followed her cat being involved in a fight with another one. She then realized that she was afraid of only one particular cat, and there was no generalization in this episode.

Throughout the treatment both direct suggestion and reassurance have been avoided. Interviews both by the psychologist and by the psychiatrist, have been confined to explaining the procedure, administering the stimuli, and assessing the position reached.

In this study there was no training in relaxation, and the presentation of anxiety-producing material was entirely *in vivo*. It was thus typical of the Maudsley approach: the follower of Wolpe would probably have trained the woman in relaxation first, and would have asked her to imagine various encounters with cats, rather than actually producing furs, pictures of cats, toy cats and real cats, etc. Nevertheless, it will be seen that the method worked very well, and except for the fact that it is sometimes much more convenient to deal with stimuli in imagination rather than in reality, it seems likely that *in vivo* desensitization has certain advantages. When stimuli have been desensitized in the imagination, there is still the step to be taken of generalizing from imagination to reality; this is avoided in the case of *in vivo* desensitization.

Let us next look at a case which typifies Wolpe's method more directly. This is a case treated by a Dr B. Ashen of the Ontario Hospital in Canada. It concerns a twenty-seven-year-old sales administrator who was suffering from a phobic fear of atomic attack. This phobia had generalized to anything connected with news of the international situation, and consequently he avoided radio, television, movies, newspapers and conversations. To escape his phobia, he travelled from England, where he had lived, to Canada, only to seek psychiatric help in the end. He was treated by a psychiatrist for two years, but the symptoms steadily got worse and he began to drink heavily to allay his anxiety. This resulted in the loss of his job and, with his fear increasing, he avoided all contact with persons and spent much of the day with the covers over his head. Suicidal ideas and an overdose of sleeping pills finally brought about certification to a mental hospital. There he was given electric shock treatments, but this only sent him back to seek escape in alcohol. His phobia placed such restrictions on his marriage that his wife was contemplating separation. This was the problem presented for treatment.

First the patient was trained in intensive muscle relaxation, and at the same time anxiety hierarchies were constructed; these were made up from the knowledge of the patient's history, and through questionnaires and interviews. The hierarchy concerning radio and television programmes, for instance, would start at the bottom with 'seeing radio and television sets in a store'. Then would come 'hearing a musical programme', then 'seeing a play on television'. The next step would be hearing an announcement of the regular news programme, and one further step up, hearing on the radio: 'We interrupt this programme to bring you a special bulletin.' Near the top would be 'going to a movie with wife, knowing there is to be a news cast', and right at the top 'turning on the radio to hear the news'. A similar series was constructed for newspaper buying, and for other aspects of his generalized fears.

In the actual desensitization programme the patient was told: 'You will now imagine a number of scenes very clearly and calmly. The scenes may not at all disturb your state of relaxation but if by any chance you feel disturbed you may indicate this to me by raising your finger an inch or so.' (A neutral stimulus would then be presented such as standing on a street corner in Toronto.) The scene would be presented for approximately five seconds and then the patient would again be instructed to relax. The least disturbing item on the newspaper hierarchy and on the radio and television hierarchy would then be presented. The patient indicated no disturbance in the actual event, and the session was ended with instructions to continue practising relax-

ations. On subsequent occasions items higher in the hierarchy
were presented, care always being taken that the patient was in a
deep state of relaxation, and that he had tolerated previous items
for ten seconds or so without signalling that they disturbed him in
any way. After thirteen desensitization sessions the patient
reported that he was listening to radio and television without
anxiety. He was allowed to go home for a weekend and reported
that he had gone to a movie with his wife. After a few more
sessions the patient was able of his own volition to turn on news
broadcasts and listen to them without evidence of anxiety. His
wife reported that he was a 'changed' person, and was able to go
out with her to the movies and visit friends. Three months
following treatment the patient reported no relapse. His wife in-
formed the psychologist who carried out the treatment that he
was in excellent health, better than he had been since she had
known him, and even though he had been unable to find another
job, he suffered no anxiety or depression and remained in excellent spirits.

Note three things about this case history. In the first place there
was a complete cure. In the second place the cure was achieved in
a very small number of sessions. And in the third place the cure
was not followed by relapse or symptom substitution, but rather
by a general improvement in the state of the patient. This should
be contrasted with the two years of treatment by psychotherapy
which only led to a worsening of his symptoms. This case is fairly
typical of a desensitization treatment by Wolpe's methods both
with respect to the way it was carried out, and also the outcome.

One further case may be of interest, if only in order to show
the extraordinary variety of different types of neurotic disorders
which can be treated by means of desensitization. The case concerns an intelligent twenty-five-year-old girl with an obsessional
personality who developed a phobia about broken glass around
which a large number of obsessional-compulsive and other symptoms were elaborated. The case was treated and described by Dr
M. T. Haslam of the Royal Victoria Infirmary in Newcastle,
England. The patient was first admitted to hospital at the age of
nineteen. Her main complaint at the time was of being unable to
face people. There was a long history of mild obsessional
behaviour which had first shown itself as a compulsive reading of
the Bible. She had an irrational fear of broken glass which had

originated in an episode when she was eighteen, when her father had been eating some jam which had some broken glass in it and badly cut his mouth. (This may be considered the original conditioning situation, interacting with a personality high on emotionality-neuroticism and very introverted.) She showed considerable depression, reactive to her compulsive symptoms which were upsetting her ability to lead a normal life. She showed extensive compulsive rituals revolving around searching for broken glass and also some compulsive washing symptoms.

Psychiatric treatment for this poor girl was rather horrific. She was given electroshock treatment but did not improve. Insulin coma therapy was also given, but had no lasting effects. Over the next four years she was admitted to hospital ten times for periods varying from a few days to five months, being again given electroshock and various drugs. In spite of all these treatments she continued to have an irrational fear of broken glass, and this fear gradually spread so that she would search everything she used, touched or ate, for broken glass. She checked every article of clothing to make sure no glass was hidden in it and had to repeat this ritual many times, getting only temporary reassurance each time. She recognized the irrationality of this behaviour but could not control it. If she tried to control it, this led to mounting tension, until she eventually gave in and repeated the ritual.

Marriage and having a baby exacerbated her obsessional and phobic symptoms. She could not cope with looking after the baby, because her compulsive searching for glass made her so slow that she was unable to give it adequate attention. This led to considerable friction between herself and her husband who even attempted to control her symptoms by using force, with the expected worsening of an already sorry state of affairs. She became depressed, obsessional and strongly phobic. Finally she underwent leucotomy, the brain operation in which the strands linking the prefrontal area with the rest of the cortex are severed. This led to a brief amelioration of the symptoms but they returned in full extent after three months. There was now talk of the baby being adopted and her husband considered leaving her. A further course of electroshock proved to be of no avail. It was at this stage that desensitization was attempted.

The therapist formulated the hypothesis that her depression and ritualistic behaviour all derived from a basic fear of being cut by broken glass, which might be in anything with which she came in contact. This had extended to include such things as tinsel and granulated sugar, since these looked similar to little bits of broken glass and might also conceal it without anyone noticing. The therapist decided to take sugar, as being only mildly productive of fear, as a starting point for reciprocal inhibition procedures. This was a convenient substance since it could be incorporated within a hunger-drive-reduction technique to reduce her anxiety. Treatment was commenced as follows. The patient was given no breakfast and no food until lunchtime. One hour before lunch she was given a small dose of tranquillising drug and at 12.30 she was given half a grapefruit (a food which she enjoyed, but which more or less demanded sugar if it were to be eaten). She was offered sugar with it. The therapist joined her in this meal, and having previously established a good rapport, this also contributed to reducing any anxiety present. She and the therapist then ate the rest of their lunch. The first session passed with minimal anxiety being shown.

This basic procedure was repeated each day, but on the third day the therapist contrived to spill a little sugar on the table which he carefully picked up on a damp finger and ate during the meal. This initially produced a little stress, but this passed off. On the next day the patient was encouraged to try to do this also, and after a little hesitation, did so. Some broken glass was introduced into the room on the next day in a bottle, and placed on the table nearest the patient while she was eating a sugared grapefruit. Over the next two or three sessions the broken glass was gradually brought nearer to the patient, and by the eighth session she was able to handle pieces of broken glass while eating her meal. It was noticed that as her confidence in this direction increased, her fears of imaginary broken glass in clothes and other places diminished, and her obsessional-compulsive rituals markedly lessened.

At the twelfth session the therapist suggested after the meal that they should go and move some broken glass from the hospital tennis court, which he had noticed earlier to be present. The patient was intitially reluctant to do this, but with encouragement eventually agreed and helped in the job. This achievement pleased her considerably, and she returned to the hospital very confident, carrying with her a piece of glass which she presented to the hitherto rather sceptical ward sister. Shortly after this she had a weekend at home, and afterwards requested her discharge. This was agreed to with reluctance as it was felt that it was still rather too early for her to go home. She had had only fourteen deconditioning sessions. However she was discharged.

Since this time she has been followed up intermittently, and nearly a year later remained symptom free. She was coping with the housework and had just had another baby without relapse. She occasionally showed obsessional traits when under stress, but her phobic symptoms had not returned and she was confident about the future. It should be noted that in the previous five years the longest period that this girl had had out of hospital had been four months, and at no time had she been symptom free.

Noteworthy about this case are two things. The first is that a number of quite extreme psychiatric procedures, such as electroshock and leucotomy, had entirely failed to have any effect on the patient. The second that a very short period of desensitization cured completely an extremely firmly established and malignant disorder. It may be noted that in this case *in vivo* desensitization was used, rather than having recourse to imaginary evocation of feared scenes and objects. Note also the use made by the therapist of modelling or imitation procedures, as when he showed the patient how to pick up the sugar on a damp finger and eat it.

The literature is full of case histories of this kind, and the reader may ask whether they give an accurate picture of the success rate which can be expected from desensitization. At this point, let us merely say that desensitization has been shown to be much more effective than classical methods of psychotherapy; we will later on discuss the effectiveness of this and other methods of behaviour therapy in more detail. For the present, and before turning to another method of treatment, namely that of 'flooding', which we have also already encountered in our discussion of animal analogues of neurosis and treatment, a few words may be said about the treatment by desensitization of sexual problems like impotence, lack of orgasm, frigidity and the like. A detailed discussion, in terms intelligible to the layman, has been given by P. and R. Gillan in their book. *Sex Therapy Today*. They explain in detail how anxiety can cause these psychophysiological symptoms, and how through desensitization such conditioned fear reactions can be eliminated. One major fear which is not infrequent in men and women is that of not coming up to expectation in their sexual 'performance'; this fear is a kind of self-fulfilling prophecy, in that the fear itself causes the failure which is feared. The cure is essentially produced by getting the patient to indulge in a series of graded 'pleasuring' encounters with wife, girl-friend or surrogate wife in which intercourse is actually forbidden and the stress is on receiving and giving pleasure through sexual play. By thus removing the fear of 'performance' failure, better adjustment is actually produced, and this, under skilful guidance, carries over into more advanced love-making and intercourse. Success in these disorders by psychotherapy has never been good; the original work of Masters and Johnson gave rather better results, and in recent years greater experience in this work has lifted the success rate to quite respectable figures. No more will be claimed at this moment, and no detailed figures will be given as the needed control figures are not available; a proper clinical trial, incorporating non-treated controls and patients treated only with psychotherapy, is urgently needed to increase one's confidence in these techniques which by common consent work much better than older methods, but which still require proper scientific support in specially designed experiments.

A last point needs to be made in connection with desensitization. Many patients complain of vague, unspecified feelings of fear and anxiety (sometimes called 'free-floating anxiety'). These seem to have no local habitation and no name, and may consequently be difficult to treat. What is usually found is that in these cases there are in fact several or even many conditioned stimuli which set off the conditioned fear response; these stimuli may be so numerous that the patient has difficulty in locating them. A lengthy discussion may be necessary to identify the problem areas, and then the therapist can begin to desensitize each particular conditioned stimulus. It is usually found that after desensitizing one or two of these stimuli, the rest decline in strength of anxiety response anyway, and are much easier to cure. Contrary to what one might have thought at first, some of these 'free-floating anxieties' are easier to treat than some apparently quite simple and straightforward phobic responses, such as agoraphobia. One's first impression can often be extremely misleading, particularly as patients do not always tell the therapists the whole truth. Quite frequently the major fear objects or situations are not even mentioned in the initial interviews, and are only unearthed later on. The task of the therapist is very much like that of a detective, or an experimenter. He has to put together a theory of what has happened from fragmentary data, unreliable witnesses and clever hunches which may be difficult to check. The fact that he is so often successful speaks well for his investigative ability.

Flooding

At first sight, the technique of 'flooding' – exposing the patient to the conditioned stimulus in its full strength right from the beginning – would seem to contradict the rule laid down for desensitization that the first step should be of a relatively innocuous experience, encountering a stimulus which produces only minimal anxiety. Another rule of desensitization, that no step should be allowed on the desensitization hierarchy which produces any great show of emotion also seems to be contradicted by the 'flooding' type of therapy. This contradiction may account for the fact that in the early work on flooding it was often found that the procedure not only failed to improve the status of the patient, but actually made him worse.

This observation is in good agreement with the theory of incubation, the hypothesis that the conditioned stimulus, when presented without reinforcement, would under certain circumstances lead to an increase in the fear/anxiety reactions already observed. Yet we have seen in the case of the dogs in the shuttlebox who were prevented from jumping over the hurdle, that response prevention, coupled with the production of the conditioned stimulus, can lead to a cure, and as we shall see shortly, this is also true in human neurosis. What is responsible for this paradox? Specially designed animal experiments have shown that the answer lies in the *duration* of exposure. When the exposure only lasts for a short time, then the anxiety reaction is enhanced ('incubation'). When the period of exposure is relatively lengthy, however, as was the case with the dogs in the shuttlebox, and as is now the case in clinical trials using 'flooding', then an original enhancement of the anxiety reaction is followed by a gradual decrease. Thus duration of exposure is crucial in these experiments, and also in clinical work.

This fact might also account for the observation that casual encounters with the feared objects, far from producing extinction of his fears in the neurotic, may actually lead to a worsening of his symptoms. Such casual encounters are usually terminated as quickly as possible by the neurotic, and are therefore only very short in duration, producing an enhancement of the neurotic reaction rather than a cure. This also agrees well with observation.

The first case to be discussed was treated by Drs R. Hodgson and S. Rachman. The patient had developed some obsessive-compulsive behaviour patterns during adolescence but did not seek psychological assistance until the age of twenty, when he was admitted to a psychiatric hospital suffering from a marked obsessional disorder. He had been dismissed from his job as a result of excessive washing rituals which interfered with his working capacity and occupied the greater part of his day. Other complaints were persistent and intrusive fears of contamination by dirt, and he displayed extensive avoidance-behaviour patterns. He was treated with drugs and supportive therapy but no improvements resulted, and after several hospital admissions a modified leucotomy was carried out, the operation being followed by the reduction of tension but no improvement in his obsessional and compulsive behaviour. Finally he was being considered for a second leucotomy, but it was decided to use desensitization treatment instead. During his treatment he was asked to imagine aversive, contaminating stimuli while relaxed, but improvement was not sufficient to constitute a cure. Then, over a four and a half month period, response prevention or flooding treatment was carried out, including also some modelling.

The patient spent almost five hours a day on his compulsive activities, experiencing particular difficulties over elimination. Before urinating or defecating he had to undress; after elimination he had to wash intensively, and frequently take showers or baths (up to five a day). He also displayed extensive and elaborate avoidance behaviour (for example, he never touched the floor, or grass, or door handles or various other things). Readers may get the idea of the nature of the washing ritual from a brief passage written by the patient in self-description:

In the toilet I wash my hands once under the tap with soap

then wash the sink out and fill it up with hot water. I then wash my hands and arms, rinse them, then wash my face. Then I wash my hands again, dry my hands and face, undo the toilet door with a paper towel then pull up my trouser zip and wash my hands and arms again taking about the same time. At all costs I must not contact any item of the toilet or sink — basin — or handle or any part of clothing after washing my hands for fear of contamination. If clothing becomes in contact with any of the above items, anything this item becomes in contact with also becomes contaminated, and so it carries on. As a rule I use my own soap. Back at the bedroom I wash my hands again, the periods before going to the toilet and after cause great worry and quite often upset me for the rest of the day.

The aim of the treatment, of course, was the extinction of maladaptive autonomic responses to dirt and excreta, and the extinction of the motor avoidance responses (for example, excessive washing). A special test was devised to measure the amount of improvement: this consisted of a number of specimens of substances which the patient could not touch prior to treatment. This avoidance test was carried out by putting out a small dish of marmalade, a jar of cigarette ash, a tin of mud, a small bottle of urine and a smear of dog excrement on a table and determining how near the patient could get to each, and whether he would be able to handle each of these contaminating items. The score obtained by adding together his distances from all the objects showed that a distance of 211 centimetres could be observed at regular intervals during the pre-treatment phase.

The major part of the treatment consisted of modelling and response prevention. The patient was asked to watch while the therapist touched the items in the avoidance test; after that he attempted to touch them himself. This was a gradual process; for instance the mud and the excrement were initially touched through a piece of paper. After watching the therapist touch the items, the patient was encouraged, but never forced, to imitate this approach behaviour. Inevitably, these sessions incorporated some period of response prevention, the patient being unable to wash his hands immediately after each attempt.

After session 15 the patient was touching the marmalade, ash and mud; during session 21 he touched the urine and during session 23 he touched the smear of excrement. After session 19 the patient began to report, for the first time, that he was noticing an improvement outside the experimental situation. This improvement continued and towards the end of the treatment the patient spent half an hour touching the smear of excrement, without washing his hands afterwards. This period of response prevention was progressively increased until it reached three hours.

During the next two months, the treatment procedure of 'modelling and response prevention' was carried out in and around the ward, in order to generalize the improvement from the experimental room to the outer world. Each day between 10.00 a.m. and 12.00 noon the patient observed the therapist touching and handling dirty objects, participated himself and was required to refrain from washing his hands or any part of his body or clothes. The patient and the therapist-model carried out activities like rubbing both hands on the floor; kneeling and sitting on the floor; rubbing coffee, chocolate, orange juice into his hands and then touching his face and clothes; touching a variety of dirty objects; sitting and lying on the grass; sitting on dirty chairs. These activities were followed by normal behaviour, such as smoking, eating, conversation and playing games, with the aim of facilitating extinction.

At the end of the treatment the patient succeeded in touching all the five substances which constituted the 'test', without having to wash his hands. There was a steady decline for both washing and toilet times over the whole treatment period, washing frequency for instance decreasing from fifteen times a day to twice a day, reflecting the total elimination of compulsive washing following chance contact with 'dirty' or 'contaminated' objects. At the end of the treatment the patient washed 87 per cent less frequently than before treatment, and spent 70 per cent less time on this behaviour.

After discharge the patient obtained a job and after six months follow-up reported he was able to maintain the job, and that there had been no relapse; the time spent going to the toilet and washing, and the frequency of occurrence, were very similar to those observed at discharge. Two years after treatment a letter of thanks was received from the patient's mother which concluded: 'He was married last September and has bought a house. He and his wife have settled in well, and it is a pleasure to call on them and see him gardening and doing various odd jobs around the house. This is a thing we would have thought impossible a few years ago.' Here is an interesting case in which the flooding and modelling procedures worked very well, but where desensitization only had a relatively mild success although even that was considerably better than the effects of orthodox psychiatric treatment administered previously.

As another example of the use of 'flooding' procedures, let us look at a group of three cases treated by Dr J. C. Boulougouris of the Athens University Medical School in Greece. The first case was that of a fifty-year-old woman severely disabled by excessive washing. Cleaning rituals were elicited in her by the fear of being contaminated by objects related to death, funerals and dirt. She avoided shaking hands with people who were holding money. Her symptoms had been present since her marriage twenty-five years earlier but over the past two years she had stayed at home all the time because of her fears that members of her family might go into the kitchen or touch objects in the house without washing. She was also unable to travel on account of her fear that somebody might touch her. Her neck was held in a flexed position.

Case two was that of a lawyer aged thirty-one who had had fears of being contaminated by syphilis since the age of eighteen. He used to avoid holding money or shaking hands with people who might have been contaminated by syphilis, and had to wash his hands many times. He kept one special suit and one pair of shoes for outdoor wear only and he did not allow his wife to touch his belongings or to enter his special changing room in his flat. Over the past year he avoided going to his office or having visitors to his house. Case three was that of a man aged thirty-four who had had rituals over the past nine years, consisting of passing through the same passages and repeatedly touching specific objects at the restaurant where he worked. He also had to dress himself by putting his clothes on and off in the same order each time. Walking and driving in the town was a major problem for him because he had to follow specific directions and use only a limited number of streets.

All these patients were treated by means of 'flooding', and assessments made of their state before and after treatment, and one, three, six and nine months later. These assessments were made by the patients themselves, by the therapist and also by an independent assessor, although this last person did not judge the follow-up results. Assessments were made of the main obsessions, of free-floating anxiety and of depression on rating scales of five points, with five indicating maximum pathology.

As an example of the treatment let us take the lawyer who was afraid of being contaminated by syphilis. He had, in all, twelve sessions (five fantasy, seven combined fantasy and practice). Marked improvement began soon after the fifth session. During the practice phase of this session the patient was taken to a hospital for venereal diseases. He was reluctant to walk through, but after firm assistance and physical pressure while he was in the hospital grounds, he started to cough continuously and became breathless and pale. He demanded his return to a safe place outside the hospital, but the therapist continued to challenge him and make him enter the hospital, touching the outside door and going into the ward and shaking hands with a syphilitic patient. The coughing and breathlessness started to subside, and the patient spontaneously said: 'I am coughing just like twelve years ago while I was in a chest clinic for tuberculosis, and I remember that in the same ward was a syphilitic patient too; it was a terrifying experience for me, I was afraid of syphilitic contamination.' A marked improvement resulted from that session; he returned to his office, went many times to the hospital, stopped washing his hands and led a happy and sociable life.

The first patient had nine sessions in all, the third patient six. Results can be seen in Figure 8, which shows the patients' ratings, the therapist's ratings and the assessor's ratings for total obsessions, free-floating anxiety and depression. It will be seen that there is a marked decrease in all these, and that this is maintained over the follow-up period. Clearly the remarkably short treatment produced an almost complete remission of the symptoms of which the patients were complaining. In these cases there was no attempt to use modelling in addition to the 'flooding' procedure.

These methods of flooding, response prevention or 'implosion', as they have variously been called, seem to be of particular use in connection with obsessive-compulsive disorders. This is particularly important because these disorders have proved

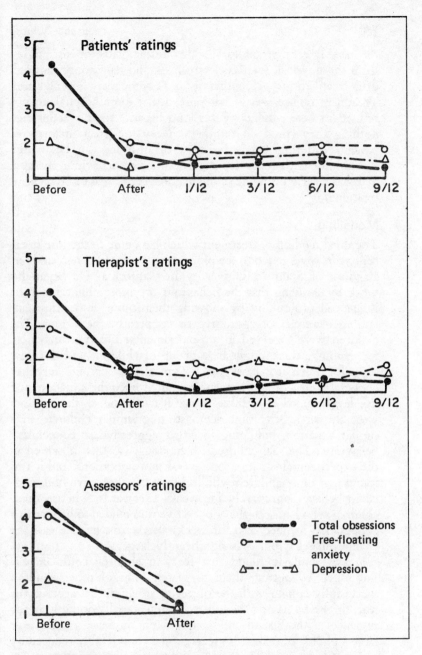

FIGURE 8
Effects of 'flooding' type treatment on three obsessive-
compulsive patients. (The ratings are the averages for
the three patients.)

remarkably recalcitrant to all other forms of treatment ranging from the physical, such as electroshock and leucotomy, through drug treatment, to psychotherapy and psychoanalysis of all kinds. Treatment failure was so widespread that some hospitals in fact refused to take patients of this kind because there was little or nothing they could do for them. Now the great majority of patients suffering from this type of disorder can be treated successfully with relatively short sessions of behaviour therapy. This has clearly been one of the major success areas of this type of treatment.

Modelling

The third method of treatment which has come to the fore in recent years owes much to the pioneering work of Professor Albert Bandura of Stanford University in California. He began his work by showing that the behaviour of young children can be influenced profoundly by showing them quite short films containing examples of aggressive or cooperative behaviour. The children were observed in an experimental situation in which, for example, there might be a group of children with too few toys for each to have one. Typically a certain level of cooperativeness or aggressiveness resulted from this situation, and this level tended to stabilise. Once it had done so, the children were shown a brief film demonstrating similar children, in a similar situation, indulging in either aggressive or cooperative behaviour. The real children's behaviour was then observed in the experimental situation on several more occasions, and it was found that those children who had seen the aggressive film tended to behave aggressively for weeks afterwards, whereas those children who had seen the cooperative film tended to behave in a cooperative manner, also for weeks afterwards. In each case the change in behaviour was significantly large.

It was similarly found that fears in children could be extinguished by getting them to watch films of other children successfully coping with the object or situation that aroused the fear, or else by having the other children actually doing so in the presence of the fearful child himself. For instance a child may have a phobia of snakes; his fears can be considerably reduced by seeing a film in which another child plays with a snake, or by observing another child doing so in his presence. This method is not as simple as it sounds. There are certain rules which have to be followed. For instance the model in the film, or the person who is performing the act which is being modelled, should be as much like the child as possible. It would be fairly useless for the act to be performed by an adult, because the phobic child knows perfectly well that adults can do things that he cannot do. Similarly, it would be disadvantageous to have the fearless act performed by a child who is fearless right from the beginning; the phobic child would simply reply that he knows that some children have no such fears but they are unlike him. The best results would be obtained by having the act modelled by a child who at first shows great fear but gradually overcomes these fears and finally is shown playing with the snake; the phobic child can identify with such a model, and the effect is much enhanced in consequence.

In a typical experiment Bandura and his colleagues worked with snake phobic adults who were made to observe a graduated film depicting models engaging in progressively more threatening interactions with a large snake. The subjects of the experiment rated the degree of fear aroused in them by the model scenes initially and at each subsequent re-exposure to the same scenes. Regardless of whether they had been instructed in relaxation or not, there was a manifest decrease in fear from the beginning through each exposure right to the end. Effects on actual behaviour with snakes could be tested and it was found that the more thoroughly the fear arousal was vicariously extinguished through viewing the films, the greater was the reduction in avoidance behaviour towards the snakes, and the more generalized were the behavioural changes. In other words, viewing the films not only had the effect of lessening anxiety to the scenes portrayed in the films, but the effect was also transferred to everyday life.

An interesting case using modelling principles has been reported by Drs Hodgson and Rachman. The patient was forty-five years of age and had a thirty-year history of compulsions to be slow, meticulous and ritualistic, especially when dressing, washing, shaving, cleaning his teeth and combing his hair. As a consequence he was unable to work since most of his day was spent in ritualistic behaviour. He would rise around 8 o'clock in the morning and would not complete his washing rituals until late afternoon! Cleaning his teeth would involve 192 slow meticulous brush strokes for each application of toothpaste and for each rinse, the whole ritual taking about half an hour. Shaving took one hour every morning, and bathing would take him up to three hours with half an hour spent rinsing the bath before filling it and half an hour rinsing the bath afterwards. Every action was performed in a slow meticulous manner reminiscent of the care taken by a bomb disposal expert. During the past thirty years the patient had seen psychiatrists and had been involved in psychoanalysis for a three-year period; he had experienced psychotherapy and drug therapy and had finally been given a leucotomy at the age of forty-three. These interventions produced little change in his obsessional behaviour.

As a first step in the treatment a number of goals were determined in collaboration with the patient. These goals were things like brushing teeth in two minutes, combing hair in two minutes, shaving in ten minutes and dressing in five minutes. Most of the therapeutic sessions were directed towards speeding up his daily rituals. The patient had been performing these intricate rituals for so long that he had forgotten the normal ways of brushing his teeth, washing and dressing. Consequently the first step involved the therapist modelling the desired behaviour by demonstrating relatively normal routines of shaving, brushing teeth, washing ears and so on. This therapeutic modelling was always followed by close observation of the patient's performance, and he was given detailed advice about which segments of his rituals could be dropped out, along with encouragement, prompting and pacing. The treatment involved only fifteen hours of the psychologist's time, and the nursing staff were drawn in to help with the work. Figure 9 shows the very substantial reduction in total time spent each week on the patient's daily rituals, including taking a bath twice each week; the target was almost but not quite reached in less than four months. As a result of treatment the patient was able to take up full employment and two years after treatment is still able to get to work on time.

Fewer applications of modelling to the treatment of neurotic disorders have been published than of desensitization and flooding. More frequently modelling has been used in conjunction with other techniques, as already illustrated in one or two cases. It also seems quite likely that the large amount of con-

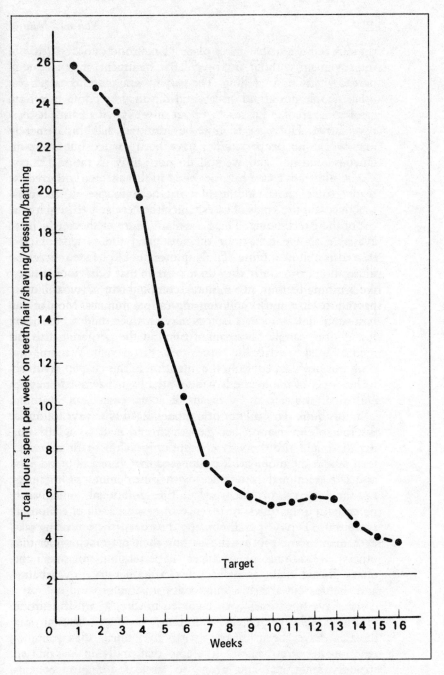

FIGURE 9
Reduction of time taken over compulsive rituals by patient
after 'modelling' type treatment.

tinuous remission that takes place in neurotic disorders (that is, improvement without any psychiatric treatment) may be due in part to vicarious modelling. The patient who is afraid of cats sees other people not afraid of cats and this may help him in certain cases to overcome his fear without any explicit treatment by a psychiatrist. However it must be admitted that this is merely guesswork; no proper studies have been carried out on spontaneous remission and we still do not know its rationale.

The illustrative case histories cited in this chapter will give the reader some understanding of what behaviourists do in actual practice, and the kinds of cases which they are able to help by the use of these techniques. There are many more methods which are available to the behaviour therapist, and the variety of cases treated is almost infinite. Those quoted should be seen merely as illustrations; obviously they do not prove that behaviour therapy works, nor do they prove that it works better than any other procedure. It is well known in clinical practice that spontaneous remission and accidental factors may produce sudden cures, and just quoting single cases cannot rule out the possibility that the method used to effect the cure is in fact irrelevant. We shall deal with this problem later on; the intention in this chapter is merely to list some of the methods widely used by behaviour therapists, and to illustrate them by means of actual cases.

In this book we shall not deal in any detail with psychosomatic disorders. The relation between them and neurosis is little understood, and also the very concept of 'psychosomatic disorders' is in flux at the moment. It is supposed that disorders of this kind associate emotional disturbances with some demonstrable damage in the organs of the body, the emotional disturbances precipitating the onset, recurrence or exacerbation of the bodily symptoms. Typical psychosomatic disorders (there is no general agreement, some psychiatrists casting their net much wider than others) are asthma, peptic ulcer, hypertension, migraine, coronary disease, diabetes mellitus, urticaria, menstrual disturbances and rheumatoid arthritis. Pulmonary tuberculosis and ulcerative colitis have sometimes been included in the list, which is by no means an inclusive one, and even lung cancer and other physical diseases have been linked with individual differences in emotional expressiveness. It seems that individuals who are strongly emotional and prone to anxiety are also prone to

develop these psychosomatic disorders, but the evidence is poor
on the whole, and it is certain that while in some people there
may be an emotional component in these disorders, in others they
may be purely medical conditions.

Of the methods used by behaviour therapists, two have shown
some promise in relation to psychosomatic disorders. An example
will demonstrate the methods and their effectiveness. The symptom treated was 'severe headaches', and the treatments were administered by Drs D. Cox, A. Freundlich and R. Meyer, of the
University of Louisville Psychology Clinic. One group of
patients was given a dummy tablet as a placebo. They were told
that this was a peripheral-acting time-release muscle-relaxant
known to be effective. Another group was taught the techniques
of muscle relaxation; after eight sessions of this they were told to
use the techniques as soon as the headache began. The third
group was given a course in 'biofeedback', a technique which
uses electric recording devices to measure the functioning of
various bodily systems, in this case the muscular system, and present the results to the patient who is then encouraged to use this
feedback in helping him to produce changes in the system – in
this case, to relax. The training consisted in teaching the subjects
to relax the frontalis muscles (the muscles in the forehead which
are usually tense during a headache). Electrodes attached to the
patients' foreheads produced bleeps according to how tense the
muscles were. Relaxation caused the bleeps to subside. After
three practice sessions, these subjects too were instructed to begin
to apply their relaxing skills at the first sign of a headache, but
they also received a further five sessions of practice and training.

The subjects recorded and rated their headaches in headache
diaries and the results are shown in Figure 10. It will be seen that
there was a marked improvement in the intensity of the
headaches experienced by the treatment groups, as compared
with the placebo group, although even that group improved
somewhat – presumably the result of suggestibility. It should be
noted that these headaches can be quite debilitating. Of the eight
subjects in the placebo group, two had to leave their harassing
jobs, another sought relaxation training, one had filed for
divorce, a fifth went into hospital, and a sixth was undergoing
chiropractice massages for his headaches. All this took place dur-

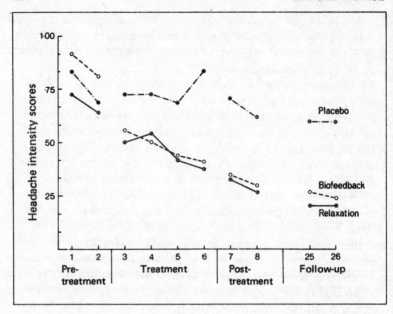

FIGURE 10
Effects on frequency of headaches of three types
of treatment.

ing the four months between post-treatment and follow-up; no
such upset befell the other groups.

In this example, biofeedback did no better than simple relaxation, possibly because we know pretty well how tense our
muscles are, and the feedback does not give us additional information. However, in other cases this may not be so, and biofeedback works quite well. One example is the facilitation of penile
erection through feedback. This has been used in males having
sexual difficulties; the practice is to show them explicit erotic
films and measure the amount of erection experienced by means
of a kind of strain gauge. Without this feedback men are apparently not very good at estimating the erectile results of the
episodes shown on the film, and there is little improvement; but
when the amount of erection is shown on a dial, using the strain
gauge as a transducer, there is an immediate and highly significant rise. We shall not discuss biofeedback further in this book,
primarily because many of the experiments using this method

have not been found possible to replicate. In the future this method may be found very useful, particularly in relation to certain psychosomatic disorders, but the time is not yet.

An interesting early example of biofeedback, long antedating the current band-wagon of applications, was carried out in our laboratories in 1954 by Professor H. Gwynne Jones. The case of the dancing girl is of particular interest because the feedback provided was in fact false, and it was this intentional error which led to recovery. The patient, a young woman of twenty-three years, was admitted to hospital as a day-patient for investigation and treatment. She complained of frequency of urination with associated secondary fears and general lack of confidence – she urinated so frequently that it made her otherwise very successful stage work as a dancer quite impossible, leading to the other consequences noted above. She was found to pass urine every thirty minutes or so, with abdominal pains. There was evidence of autonomic imbalance in that her limbs were at times very cold, at other times warm, and that she sweated copiously. No physical cause of abnormality was found, and she was diagnosed as suffering from hysterical urinary frequency – a rather unhelpful diagnosis! Psychotherapy and general hospital treatment provided no relief.

Behaviour therapy using biofeedback was tried, using a method of conditioning urinary frequency first established by the Russian physiologist K. M. Bykov. A manometer (an instrument for measuring the pressure of a gas or fluid) was constructed, fitted with a scale in arbitrary units, and connected, by means of an inconspicuous tap, to a syringe; this created a back pressure and decreased the reading on the scale without the patient's knowledge. By means of the apparatus, with appropriate arrangements of the clips and taps, varying volumes of sterile saline solution could be introduced into the patient's bladder, true or decreased readings could be taken at any stage of the patient's bladder pressure, and the patient's bladder could be voluntarily evacuated, the outflow being measured in a cylinder. In use the manometer was placed at bladder height and immediately before the patient where she could read the scale.

In the patient, so it was found, the urge to urinate occurred at relatively low bladder volumes and pressures; furthermore, her bladder musculature maintained abnormally high bladder pressure at abnormally low bladder volumes. The conditioning treatment made use of the fact that the patient felt a strong urge to urinate when the manometer reading reached a level of 7 arbitrary units (roughly corresponding to 550 ml. of fluid.) Introducing fluid into the bladder, and operating the back pressure to lower the readings, she was persuaded to accept higher and higher amounts of fluid, under the mistaken impression that she had not yet reached her usual maximum when in fact she had exceeded it. Gradually, by a skilful mixture of true and faked readings, the patient was brought to ever higher levels, and also to a realization that she could tolerate these higher levels without urinating. The cure of this symptom in the non-stressful environment of the hospital was followed by a graded re-education programme before effective relief from the symptoms in normal life situations was achieved. The treatment was successful, and fifteen months after her discharge, her private physician reported that she had remained free of symptoms and had recently married with apparent success.

This last statement may be relevant because the psychiatric history revealed certain sexual events which might have been instrumental in causing the hysterical (or psychosomatic) complaint. At the age of seventeen she had had intercourse with a young man; this caused her much anxiety, and the *coitus interruptus* they practised was unpleasant for her. Her urinary frequency dated from that time and within a year caused her acute embarrassment. It is likely that these events provided the unconditioned stimuli, and that the cure for her urinary frequency also lowered her sexual anxieties sufficiently for normal sexual relations to be established. It is interesting to contemplate the kind of treatment this girl would have received from a psychoanalyst, with the likely outcome of retaining her symptom but knowing a great deal more about her unconscious (and probably imaginary) sex life, and her unconscious (and equally imaginary) Elektra complexes.

It is sometimes claimed that Freud 'discovered' the existence of psychosomatic diseases. Like so many other claims, this one is without foundation. As early as 1843, William Sweetser remarked that 'few, we imagine, have formed any adequate estimate of the sum of bodily ill which originates in the mind'. Similarly, the German psychiatrist Heinroth used the concept in 1815, and long before that Plutarch quoted the established wisdom of Greek physicians: 'If the body sued the mind for damages, the mind would be found to have been a ruinous tenant for its landlord.' As in relation to so many other 'discoveries' of the Freudians, one is forced to say that what is true in them is not new, and what is new is not true. Even the 'unconscious', of course, has a history reaching back over the centuries, anticipating all the possibly valid claims made for it nowadays.

5 Asocial and Antisocial Behaviour

The causes of criminality

We have hitherto dealt entirely with the so-called dysthymic disorders – *conditioned emotional responses which are maladaptive* and which occur primarily in introverted, high N people genetically predisposed to form such conditioned responses. However, as C.G. Jung was the first to point out, introverts are not the only ones to show neurotic, unstable, maladaptive responses; so do extraverts, although their behaviour is quite different from that of introverts. Jung suggested that neurotic introverts show *psychasthenic* reactions, whereas extraverts manifest *hysterical* symptoms. This is partly true; certainly patients with hysterical personalities, who are histrionic, unreliable, and with violent mood changes, tend to score much more extraverted on personality inventories than do psychasthenics or dysthymics. (The term 'psychasthenia' is obsolete, but it refers to pretty much the same range of symptoms as does dysthymia.)

Hysteria was frequently diagnosed and found in the days of the first world war and before, but nowadays it has become a rarity. The typical extraverted disorders are the so-called 'personality disorders' and psychopathy, that is to say asocial or antisocial behaviour without manifestations of guilt or conscience. Psychopathy and personality disorders are of course closely related to criminality, although there is no one-to-one correspondence. (The term 'psychopathy', or 'sociopathy' as it is often called in the United States, is poorly understood by psychiatrists. There are probably different kinds of psychopath, sometimes called primary and secondary. It would be impossible here to go into the details of the difference, or their relation to psychosis or neurosis, but primary psychopaths are probably nearer to the psychotic, secondary psychopaths to the neurotic variety of abnormality.)

Criminals are a very heterogeneous group, and although many

140

criminals are psychopaths, others are not. Neither are all psychopaths criminals; their antisocial behaviour might come close to bringing them into conflict with the law, but they may never cross the threshold, or else they may be lucky in not being reported, detected, or convicted. The terms 'personality disorder' and 'psychopathy' are often used interchangeably, although perhaps the term psychopath (or the more modern term sociopath) denotes a rather more advanced state of antisocial behaviour.

Many people, including psychiatrists, would probably jib at describing criminals as neurotics, although most would probably agree that psychopaths and behaviour disorders should be so classified. Justification for doing so rests on two facts. The first is the close association between personality disorders and psychopathy, on the one side, and criminal behaviour on the other. The second justification lies in the fact that criminals, behaviour disorders, psychopaths and others who indulge in frequent antisocial behaviour tend to have high scores on N – just about as high as do dysthymic neurotics in many cases. This connection with personality is very important for anyone trying to understand the dynamics of antisocial and criminal behaviour. As already mentioned, neurotics tend to come from the *melancholic quadrant*, criminals from the *choleric quadrant*, that is, neurotics tend to be introverted and high on N, whereas criminals tend to be extraverted and high on N. There is much evidence to demonstrate the validity of this statement.

The first line of evidence comes from the study of school-children. Thousands of boys and girls, both middle class and working class, and attending both comprehensive and grammar schools, have been tested with personality inventories and their degree of antisocial behaviour measured. This was done both objectively, by reference to known misdeeds at school and outside, and subjectively, by furnishing them with a list of the kinds of antisocial acts that children often or sometimes indulge in, letting them pick out those of which they themselves had been guilty. The two criteria correlate to a satisfactory degree, and both show quite high correlations with extraversion and a high degree of neuroticism. In other words, those children who behave in an antisocial fashion, whether boys or girls, tend to come from the choleric quadrant.

Similar studies have been done with adolescents, and here too there is a very distinct relationship between antisocial behaviour, this time of a more serious nature than in the case of children, and extraversion combined with a high degree of N. This relationship is found both in adolescents already incarcerated for criminal activity, and also in adolescents still at large.

With adults, literally thousands of criminals have been tested and compared with equal numbers of non-criminal members of the population, matched for age, sex and social status. The outcome has been that in practically every case the criminals have a much higher neuroticism score, and that on the whole they tend to be more extraverted. This extraversion has manifested itself, however, more in the field of impulsiveness than in that of sociability – possibly due to the fact that to a prisoner actually incarcerated for many years questions about going to parties and enjoying meeting many people may be rather meaningless! However that may be, results from children, adolescents and adults support the general view that antisocial conduct is related to extraverted personality, particularly when combined with high degrees of N.

Could it be that it is incarceration which produces the personality features, rather than the other way about? Follow-up studies of children suggest that this is not so. Sir Cyril Burt had teachers rate the personality of 763 children on extraversion and neuroticism; of these 15 per cent and 18 per cent respectively later became habitual offenders or neurotics. The follow-up of the children disclosed after some 30 years that of those who became habitual offenders, 63 per cent had been rated as high on neuroticism; 54 per cent had been rated as high on extraversion, but only 3 per cent as high on introversion. Of those who became neurotics, 59 per cent had been rated as high on neuroticism; 44 per cent had been rated high on introversion, with only 1 per cent high on extraversion. Thus we see that even the probably rather unreliable ratings made by teachers of their pupils at school can predict with surprising accuracy the later adult behaviour of these children. The concordance is surprising because luck and the unforeseeable circumstances of life must play a large part in determining whether a given person prone to crime or neurosis does in fact succumb, and other personality traits and abilities obviously also play a part in the social adjustment of the person. However that may be, the figures as they stand argue convincingly for the predetermination of later conduct, whether the criminal or neurotic, by personality. Other follow-up studies, although less convincing, have also pointed in the same direction.

Before turning to the question of how we can account for this connection between extraversion and antisocial behaviour, let us consider the problem of genetic and environmental causes. It is usually assumed by modern sociologists that crime is produced by environmental causes, among which poverty, social inequality, alienation induced by capitalist work practices, bad housing, and so on, play a large part. It is quite possible that these alleged causes do play some part in accounting for delinquency, but clearly there are considerable difficulties in accepting such arguments as convincing. In the first place, among people subjected to identical degrees of poverty and alienation, some do become criminals, others do not; similarly, among people not subjected to these conditions, some also become criminals, others do not. Clearly, there are other powerful factors in determining whether a person will or will not become a criminal. Another major difficulty lies in the fact that over the past thirty years or so social conditions in the so-called capitalist countries have improved dramatically, leading to a much higher standard of living for the poorer classes of the population, a very marked lessening of inequality of wealth, a higher standard of housing, and other advances. According to the theory, this should have led to a lessening in crime, but exactly the opposite has happened – there has been an unprecedented increase in crime over the same period. Thus the theory predicts a negative correlation between social well-being and crime, but the facts suggest a strong positive correlation. This must lower one's belief in the accuracy of the prediction, and the value of the theory as a whole.

Another reason for doubting the Marxist theory which links capitalism with crime lies in the fact that the socialist countries behind the Iron Curtain have certainly not been successful in eradicating crime, although some form of socialism has been the norm of life there for quite a long time. If personality in fact should prove to be an important factor in criminality, then we would expect criminals in communist and socialist countries to show the same kind of personality structure as do criminals in the

Western world, compared with non-criminals in these countries. Studies have actually been carried out in Hungary and Czechoslovakia in an attempt to test this hypothesis, and the outcome has been very clear-cut: criminals in communist countries as compared with non-criminals in communist countries show the same personality pattern (high neuroticism and high extraversion) as do criminals in the Western countries compared with non-criminals in the Western countries. This would be very difficult to explain in terms of an environmentalist theory, and particularly in terms of a Marxian interpretation of antisocial behaviour. (It should be noted in this context that the criminals tested in Hungary and Czechoslovakia were not political prisoners, but criminals guilty of the same kinds of crimes – burglary, robbery, etc. – as were the criminals tested in the Western world.)

The relation between personality and antisocial behaviour observed both in the West and in communist countries has also been observed in countries of the Third World, like India. It seems to be true that we may regard this relationship as invariant across many different cultures, and this suggests immediately that there are some genetic causes active in producing it. This is of course all the more likely as we have already seen that both extraversion and neuroticism are determined to a large extent by genetic factors. Is there any truth in this unpopular hypothesis? There are two lines of evidence which seem to indicate that antisocial and criminal behaviour has a strong genetic basis. The first source of evidence is the study of concordance for criminality between identical and fraternal twins. In studies of this kind, the investigator looks at a given prison population and picks out all those prisoners who are noted as having a twin; he then looks up the twin to find out whether he is an identical or fraternal twin, and also whether he is concordant for criminality or not, that is, whether he too has committed a crime. If heredity plays an important part in causing criminality, then identical twins should be concordant more frequently than fraternal twins, because they share a common heredity with the original prisoner to a much more marked extent than would a fraternal twin. There are by now ten different experiments involving over 1,000 pairs of twins, and carried out in many different countries including Germany, the Scandinavian countries and America; in all of these it has been found that the ratio of concordance for identical twins to that of fraternal twins is over four to one. In other words if a prisoner has an identical twin, that twin is over four times as likely also to have committed a crime as would a fraternal twin! This is a very large difference indeed, strongly suggestive of genetic determination.

Support for this hypothesis also comes from adoption studies. In one of these, carried out in Denmark, 57 psychopathic adoptees were compared with 57 non-psychopathic control adoptees, equated for sex, age, social class and in many cases neighbourhood of rearing and age of transfer to the adopting family; carefully defined criteria for psychopathic behaviour were used in this study. Next, the investigator examined the case records of the biological and adoptive relatives of the psychopathic and control subjects. In spite of the fact that adoption took place at an early age, there were no differences whatsoever between the adoptive families of the psychopathic and the control groups; when it came to the biological family members of these groups, however, relatives of the psychopathic boys showed an incidence of psychopathy two and a half times as great, and an incidence of mildly psychopathic behaviour also two and a half times as great, as were found in relatives of the control boys. In other words, the psychopathic boys had taken after the biological parents, not their adopted parents.

The other study was carried out in Iowa, in the United States, and here interest was not in diagnosed psychopathy but rather in actual records of crime and arrest. The investigator started off by locating 41 female criminal offenders who were inmates of a women's prison reformatory and who had given up their babies for adoption at birth. At the time of study they had produced 52 offspring, ranging in age from fifteen to forty-five years. A properly matched control group was also studied, consisting of 52 offspring from non-criminal mothers who had also been given up for adoption. It was found that the offspring of the criminal mothers had had more criminal arrests, and had also received a much greater number of convictions; these differences are fully significant statistically. Here too, therefore, the children seemed to follow their biological parents, not their adoptive parents, in spite of the fact that it was the adoptive parents who produced their environment almost from the moment of birth onwards.

All this of course merely proves the importance of genetic factors; it is not intended to suggest that environmental factors do not also play an important part. All behaviour is governed by the interaction between environment and heredity; only a fool would deny the importance of the one or the other, and claim that all behaviour was determined entirely by one set of factors alone. Difficult though it may be, the investigator must look at all the evidence and try to assess the relative importance of different elements in their contribution to a given type of behaviour, whether neurotic or criminal.

We have now seen that genetic factors contribute to the determination of criminal behaviour, and that they probably do so through personality factors. Can we account for criminal behaviour in terms of the general theory we have put forward in the third chapter? The answer to this question is in the affirmative, but we can here only delineate the theory in broad outline; for details the reader must be referred to my book *Crime and Personality*. Such a brief presentation may sound dogmatic and possibly unconvincing but pressure of space makes it impossible to go into greater detail.

We have already noted the two major points which enter into the theory I am now going to propose. The first is that extraverts condition less well and strongly than do ambiverts – people intermediate between the extremes – whereas introverts condition better and more quickly than ambiverts. We have seen that the troubles of the introvert are related to this quick, strong conditioning of emotional reactions: could it be that the troubles of the extravert may be related to his lack of conditioning facility? The answer would seem to be that they are. We all have to acquire the patterns of socialized behaviour in infancy, and quite clearly the infant cannot acquire these patterns through the exercise of reason; his intellect is simply not developed sufficiently for such intellectual learning to take place. The most plausible alternative is that we acquire a 'conscience' through a long continued process of conditioning, in which the 'naughty', 'bad', 'wicked' actions are the conditioned stimuli, and the resulting punishment and consequent feelings of pain, fear and anxiety are the unconditioned stimuli and responses respectively. Through a number of repetitions of such pairings between misdeed and punishment the child begins to form conditioned responses which lead him to react with anxiety to the contemplation of carrying out any further acts of this kind. Thus according to this theory, *conscience is a conditioned response*, or rather a whole set of conditioned responses. Introverts acquire these responses easily and quickly, and therefore tend to behave in a socialized manner; extraverts acquire them only slowly and painfully and consequently their 'conscience' is much less fully developed than that of the introvert, or even that of the ambivert. Can the process of conditioning provide a strong enough motive for behaving in a socialized manner? For an answer, let us turn to an animal experiment which will illustrate the theories here outlined.

The experiments here briefly recounted were originally carried out by Professor Richard L. Solomon and some of his colleagues at Harvard University, and later in Philadelphia, using six-months-old puppies. Later experiments have also been carried out with young children, but we shall concentrate here on the animal experiments. These were carried out in an empty room furnished with just a chair which was placed in a corner; in front of the chair were placed two small dishes. The experimenter sat in the chair, holding in his hand a rolled-up newspaper with which he could swat the puppies on the rump. Each of the puppies was deprived of food for two days and was then brought into the experimental room. In one of the dishes had been placed boiled horsemeat, which was very much liked by the puppies, whereas in the other dish was placed a much less well liked commercial dog food. The puppies usually made straight for the horsemeat, but as they touched it they were swatted by the experimenter. If one gentle blow was not enough, then the puppy was swatted again and again until he finally gave up his attempts to eat the horsemeat. Usually several further attempts were made, until finally the puppies turned to the commercial dog food, which they could eat without being swatted.

This training was carried on for several days, until the puppies had firmly learned that the horsemeat was taboo. The experimenter then turned to what was called the 'temptations testing' phase. Again the puppies were deprived of food for two days and then brought to the room, but this time with the experimenter absent. Again a choice had to be made between a dish of boiled horsemeat and a few pellets of dog food. The puppies soon gobbled up the dog food, then began to react to the large dish of horsemeat. In Solomon's words:

> Some puppies would circle the dish over and over again.
> Some puppies walked around the room with their eyes
> towards the wall, not looking at the dish. Other puppies got
> down on their bellies and slowly crawled forward, barking
> and whining. There was a large range of variability in the
> emotional behaviour of the puppies in the presence of the
> tabooed horsemeat. We measured resistance to temptation as
> the number of seconds or minutes which passed by before the
> subject ate the tabooed food.

The puppies were allowed half an hour in the experimental
room. If they did not eat the horsemeat by that time, they were
brought back to their home cages, were not fed, and, a day later,
were introduced again to the experimental room. This continued
until the puppies finally violated the taboo and ate the horsemeat,
or until they had fasted so long that they had to be fed in their
cage in order to keep them alive.

There was a very great range of resistance to temptation. The
shortest period of time it took a puppy to overcome his training
and eat the horsemeat was six minutes, and the longest period of
time was sixteen days without eating, after which time the experiment had to be stopped and the puppy fed in its own cage.
This great range of variability made it possible to test the influence of various experimental conditions on the growth of
'conscience' in these puppies. For instance, it was shown that
when the puppies were hand-fed throughout their early life by
the experimenter, they developed a conscience much more
strongly than did other animals which had been machine-fed.

Changes in the experimental situation showed that when the
puppies were swatted just when they approached the tabooed
food, they built up a high resistance to temptation. However,
when such puppies did kick over the traces, they showed no
emotional upset following the crime. On the other hand, when
the puppies were left to eat half the horsemeat before being
swatted, then one could still establish an avoidance of the
horsemeat. In the case of these puppies, however, there was much
more emotional disturbance following the crime, and these,
Solomon suggested, could be called guilt reactions. The presence
of the experimenter was not required to elicit these reactions,

although his presence seemed to intensify them when he did
finally come into the room after the 'crime' had been committed.
'Therefore we believe that the conditions for the establishment of
strong resistance to temptation as contrasted with the capacity to
experience strong guilt reactions, are a function of both the intensity of punishment and the time during the approach and con-
sumatory response sequence at which the punishment is administered.'

Solomon did not link up his results particularly with individual
differences and ease of conditioning, but he does refer to the fact
that different breeds of dogs differ very much in the ease with
which they acquire a 'conscience'. Thus for instance Shetland
sheep dogs are especially sensitive to reprimand: taboos can apparently be established in them with just one conditioning experience and are then extremely resistant to extinction. On the
other hand, he reports, Basenjis seem to be constitutional psychopaths, and it is very difficult to maintain taboos in such dogs.
All these findings, then, are in very good agreement with our
general hypothesis.

So far we have been dealing with the personality factor of extraversion. Why is it that neuroticism also plays an important
part in the genesis of criminal behaviour? The answer is to be
found in a general law we have already mentioned previously, in
connection with the establishment of dysthymic reactions. It is
widely accepted that behaviour results from habits which are activated by drives, and as a rough and ready guide we may assume
that the strength of the behaviour is determined by the multiplicative combination of drive and habit. Now, as we have
seen, fear and anxiety are strong drives, and consequently
whatever habit, neurotic or antisocial, a person or a dog or rat
may possess, this will be multiplied by the fear/anxiety drive under which he is working, to produce the actual behaviour. Now
the high N personality is obviously much more susceptible to
evocation of fear/anxiety responses, and consequently much
more likely to have a strong drive to combine with whatever
neurotic or antisocial habits he may have. Thus the extravert,
assuming him to have antisocial habits, will demonstrate these
much more strongly if he also has a high degree of N, leading
him to have frequent strong fear/anxiety drives. Again an animal
experiment may be a useful illustration of what is meant here.

In this experiment, which was carried out with rats, I laid down a law of socialization for them: they had to wait three seconds after the food had been dumped into their hopper before starting to eat. This 'law' was enforced by giving the animals a mild electric shock if they started to eat before the proper time. There are three possible reactions for animals to show, and indeed all of these reactions were shown by some animals. In the first place there is the *integrated* or normal reaction: the rat learns to wait for three seconds and then goes and eats the food in the hopper. The second is the *neurotic* reaction: the animal gets so upset and frightened that he goes and sits in the corner and does not eat at all, although it is perfectly safe to do so. The third reaction is the *psychopathic* or criminal one: the rat goes and eats the moment the food is put in the hopper, although he is being punished for it each time. We may assume that some animals genetically start off with a more introverted or dysthymic personality, others with a more extraverted or criminal personality. We now come to the crucial part of the experiment.

We had been breeding emotional and non-emotional rats for a period of many years, until we had two genetically quite distinct strains. The deduction was made from the general theory that neurotic and psychopathic responses to the situation would occur primarily among the emotional rats, whereas integrated or normal reactions would be much more prominent among the non-emotional rats. This was predicted upon the hypothesis that the high degree of emotionality of the emotional strain would multiply the neurotic or psychopathic tendencies or habits in these animals and would then lead to the respective behaviour patterns. This was found to be indeed so. Neurotic and psychopathic reactions were found almost exclusively among the emotional rats, normal or well adapted reactions among the non-emotional rats. It is always dangerous of course to argue from the behaviour of rats to that of humans, but these experiments will illustrate the way the general theory is supposed to work in the case of humans, even though we cannot necessarily accept the rat experiment as proof of its validity.

We have so far dealt with behaviours which are antisocial. There are also behaviours which are asocial, that is to say they are not criminal or directly harmful to members of the population, but nevertheless contravene the mores of that society and are therefore regarded as undesirable by many people. Homosexuality, fetishism and other sexual aberrations are among the more prominent of these activities; so are alcoholism, drug taking (where this is not actually a criminal offence) and so on. These behaviours, like antisocial behaviours, may also come to the attention of the psychiatrist, and the question arises whether behaviour therapy has any suggestions to make in this connection. The case here seems to be exactly the opposite to that presented by typical dysthymic disorders. Where the dysthymic has a number of conditioned responses which are maladaptive and which he wishes to extinguish, the criminal, the psychopath, or the person suffering from personality disorder, has *failed* to form conditioned responses which would enable him to behave in a socially approved manner. What would be needed in his case is clearly a dose of conditioning which would provide for him what he had failed to acquire previously.

This is the general principle of behaviour therapy in the type case mentioned; obviously many ethical and other problems are raised in connection with criminality, psychopathy, homosexuality, etc., which would not arise in the case of the dysthymic disorders. For one thing, the dysthymic is himself the sufferer from his neurotic disorders, and it is he who appeals to the psychiatrist for help. In the case of the criminal or the psychopath, however, it is other people who suffer and it is they who complain about the behaviour of the criminal or the psychopath. He himself is often quite satisfied with his life and his behaviour, his only complaint being that in living out his wishes and desires he comes into conflict with society and may be sent to prison, or punished in other ways. Were it not for that, he would be quite happy and contented! This of course is not universally true. Homosexuals often wish to be different, and come to the psychiatrist of their own accord; so do fetishists, alcoholics and others. Even criminals often complain that there is 'something in them' which makes them commit crimes, and that they would dearly like to get rid of this 'something'. I have had letters from prisoners to this effect. Nevertheless in the majority of cases there is pressure from society for these people to alter their behaviour; then the question arises as to the degree to which the psychiatrist should cooperate with society in enforcing its will upon people of this kind. This and other ethical problems will be discussed briefly at the end of this book; we will only hint at the existence of the problem here.

Aversion Therapy

These antisocial and psychopathic disorders, in a meaningful way, represent the opposite of dysthymic disorders and require an opposite type of therapy. What is meant by this statement? Essentially, in dysthymic disorders we are dealing with superfluous and maladaptive emotions that have to be extinguished; now we are dealing with emotional reactions that have never become conditioned. Consequently what is needed in these cases is the establishment of conditioned responses. In the case of antisocial behaviour, what we have to do is to link unpleasant, painful and fear/anxiety producing reactions with the kind of activity in question — crime, alcoholism, sexuality, fetishism, drug taking or whatever. This is the principle underlying aversion therapy and it may be illustrated by the earliest recorded case of aversion therapy. This is a story told by Plutarch about Demosthenes, who was suffering from a shoulder tic, a tendency to jerk up his shoulder spasmodically. In order to cure this tic he suspended a very sharp sword over his shoulder so that whenever the tic occurred, the shoulder jerked up against the point of the sword which pierced the skin and produced a painful unconditional stimulus. By pairing the jerk of the shoulder with the aversive puncturing of the skin, Demosthenes cured himself of his shoulder tic!

It might be objected that all methods of punishment, such as imprisonment, birching, or even simple fines employ the same principle. The crime committed is punished by inflicting upon the evil-doer undesirable consequences, in the hope that this will deter him from further evil-doing, and will act in such a way as to produce fear/anxiety responses in the future when he is contemplating further crime. There are several answers to this argument, the main one being that conditioning, as we have already noted, is very dependent on certain experimental parameters, such as accurate timing. Conditioning only takes place when the unconditioned stimulus is administered fairly shortly after the conditioned stimulus. In a typical laboratory situation the interval should not be longer than a second or so; in cases of conditioned stimuli which show the property of 'preparedness' this time may be extended a little, but not too much. Certainly the length of time which elapses between the commission of a crime, the apprehension of the culprit, the pronouncement of the sentence, and then the beginning of the punishment is far too long to allow of any ordinary type of conditioning to take place. To some mild extent conditioning may be mediated through the second signalling system, that is, through conscious thought, but this is very much weaker than conditioning proper and probably does not play a very important part in the socialization process. Certainly the evidence is pretty strong that the ordinary process of punishment does not have much effect on criminals; the criminological literature is full of evidence of recidivism which bears out this point.

We can illustrate the way that aversion therapy works by reference to alcoholism. Typically the alcoholic is placed in a room which contains a bottle of his favourite tipple. He is given a drug such as apomorphine, which has the effect of making a person sick at the stomach until he finally vomits. The psychologist monitors the bodily reactions of the patient, and just before he is overcome by nausea asks him to drink a glass of wine, or spirits, or whatever he happens to have chosen. The drink is the conditioned stimulus; the nausea and the resulting vomiting are the unconditioned responses to which the experimenter wishes to link the conditioned stimulus, so that in future the sight and feel of a drink produces the same feelings of sickness and nausea. This experiment is repeated a number of times until finally the desired effect is obtained, and the patient does feel nausea at the sight of alcoholic drinks.

This, very much over-simplified, is an account of the sort of thing that psychologists and psychiatrists have been trying to do for many years. Does it work? This is apparently a simple question, but there is no simple answer to it. In the first place the result is determined by many details of experimental procedure, such as the precise timing involved, the amount of apomorphine given, the number of conditioning trials, the personalities of the patients involved, and many other such factors which make it difficult to form any kind of generalization. Perhaps it would not be too inaccurate to state (a) that most people do produce conditioned responses of the desired kind; (b) that many people generalize these responses from the laboratory to the outer world; and (c) that a relatively small proportion of people are permanently cured in this manner. It is also unfortunately true that (d) many people apparently cured have a relapse after some time; these can be helped by a repetition of the process. Under these conditions, it is reported in the largest and best controlled series of studies that something like 50 per cent of alcoholics can be permanently cured in this manner. This is not perhaps anything like as high a figure as one might have desired, but it is well known that all methods of treatment of alcoholism are subject to relapse, and can claim only a very small number of permanent successes. Why is this so?

There are many good reasons. In the first place the treatment of alcoholism is rather unpleasant, both for the patient and also for the doctor and the nurses; nobody likes being sick at his stomach and vomiting, and nobody likes cleaning up after him! This means that usually only a minimal number of pairings of apomorphine and drink is administered, so that the amount of conditioning achieved is at a relatively low level. If we could double or treble the number of pairings, then probably the effects would be stronger. The next difficulty is that it would be inhumane, and possibly medically dangerous, to make the unconditioned response too strong; yet the effectiveness of the conditioning procedure depends to some extent on the strength of the unconditioned stimulus. This is an obvious ethical and social difficulty which besets all aspects of aversion therapy.

A third difficulty is the obvious one that all conditioned responses are subject to extinction. Inevitably the patient will come across pubs, drinks, and other stimuli which will produce only a mild, conditioned form of nausea, and consequently in many cases extinction will take place. Presumably in some cases we will also find incubation, as described in a previous chapter, and this may account for the number of successful treatments. Nevertheless, in a majority of cases extinction can be predicted to take place, and does in fact take place; thus our theoretical expectations are unfortunately borne out in fact.

There is one additional difficulty which is probably more important than those mentioned hitherto. Usually there are good reasons why a person starts drinking, and becomes an alcoholic. Alcohol is not an aphrodisiac, but a tranquillizer; it has been shown experimentally to reduce anxiety and make it more bearable. A person may become an alcoholic because he 'drowns his sorrows in alcohol'; if we now cure him of his alcohol addiction we still leave him with his sorrows, as it were, and therefore with a very strong motivation to seek solace again in drink. Furthermore, an alcoholic has reshaped his whole life in such a way that he depends for social intercourse and in many other ways on his friends who are drinking with him. Remove the alcohol and he loses not only the drink, but also the camaraderie and friendship with these people, and we have put nothing in their place. In other words although the operation is successful, the patient is by no means well. We have taken away quite successfully the craving for alcohol, but we have done nothing to remove the causes of the craving, and we have left him with a big hole in his life which we have done nothing to fill.

Clearly we must make a distinction between the aim of the experiment, which is to produce an aversive conditioned reaction to alcohol and which is successfully accomplished, and the general psychiatric aim of making a person mentally healthy and not dependent on alcohol. This requires much more than just aversion therapy; it clearly requires a removal of the fear, anxieties and depressive feelings which originally caused him to take refuge in alcohol, which might be accomplished by any of the methods of behaviour therapy already discussed. What is further required is the creation of a new mode of life which would fill in the hole left by the abandonment of his drinking cronies. Thus the general psychiatric aim is much wider than that of the rather narrow psychological experiment, and often more difficult to accomplish. Aversion therapy within the narrow framework in which it is set works remarkably well; to produce a permanent cure it has to be set in a much wider context, and this may be difficult to accomplish.

What is true of alcoholism is true of the other types of disorder we are going to discuss also. Usually the narrow psychological experiment can be carried out successfully and with predictable consequences; it is the general psychiatric management of the case which may present difficulties because the psychological experiment by itself does not change the life conditions which have led the individual into the cul-de-sac from which we are trying to rescue him. This can be done, and such bodies as Alcoholics Anonymous for instance have clearly realised the necessity for social integration and support, as have individual psychiatrists who follow up their cases and give them psychiatric support and treatment in addition to simple aversion therapy. However the important thing is that aversion therapy, if only a first step, is an essential first step as without it we could not make a proper beginning in the treatment of alcoholism and similar disorders.

Homosexuality is often treated by aversion therapy in a rather similar manner, although apomorphine and nausea is often replaced by an electric shock. The method used is pretty obvious. The patient is shown pictures of nude males; an electric shock is administered shortly afterwards, increasing in intensity until the patient pushes a button which removes the picture and the shock simultaneously. This is repeated a large number of times in order to associate the picture of nude males, and the accompanying sexual thoughts, with pain, fear and discomfort rather than with pleasurable sensations. This procedure can of course be complicated in many different ways, but essentially that is the aim of the experiment, and very frequently it succeeds in reaching this aim. Can homosexuality be 'cured' in this way? (The term 'cured' has been put in quotes because it would of course be incorrect to think of homosexuality as a disease in any way. Homosexuality is perfectly natural, in the sense that it occurs in nature, in other animals as well as in man, and while it is disapproved of in our society, or certainly used to be until quite recently, it has been approved of in other societies, such as among the Ancient Greeks. The term 'cured' is used here because the individual who comes for treatment regards homosexuality as an undesirable mode of behaviour which he wishes to get rid of; in that sense it resembles the anxieties, fears and depressions of the dysthymic, and the term 'cure' may be appropriate.)

As with alcoholism, a certain proportion of homosexuals are 'cured' by one set of conditioning experiences. Many have a relapse, and may be 'cured' permanently by another administration of the conditioning procedure. Many patients feel the effect of the procedure, but ultimately relapse completely. Homosexuality like alcoholism is quite complex, and there are implications for social relationships in the treatment which have to be taken into account. The homosexual may be actually afraid of women, and have no special skills in getting to know and bed women; thus a 'cure' leaves him incapable of forming the kinds of social relationships which are implicit in heterosexual conduct. His whole life has been built up on friendships with homosexuals, living in homosexual surroundings, clubs and so on, and if all this is now withdrawn there is again a gaping hole in his social life. For many homosexuals there is just no positive feeling of a sexual kind towards women; this again makes life impossibly difficult for them after the 'cure'. Psychologists have attempted to get over these difficulties.

One way of changing the attitude of the homosexual who is afraid of women, of course, is to treat him by a desensitization process. This has proved very effective, and in fact by itself sometimes effects a 'cure'. In order to evoke a positive reaction to women what is sometimes done is to introduce pictures of women, both clothed and nude, at the moment that the patient presses a button to stop the shock and the exposure of the pictures of nude males. In this way the picture of the woman is associated with relief from pain and thus with positive feelings. Crude as this method is, it seems to work quite well in many cases.

But most of all, what the therapist often has to do is to give the patient training in certain social skills, including that of meeting women, talking to them, and even seducing them. This may sound a very odd job for a doctor or a psychologist, but without some such training a relapse is very likely, and may even be inevitable. It will be obvious that all this raises ethical questions which are quite unusual, and which few doctors or psychologists have been trained to deal with. Nevertheless if we wish to help the homosexual who comes begging for treatment because for one reason or another he is extremely dissatisfied with his mode of living and wishes to change it, can we in all conscience refuse? We shall return to this problem later.

The treatment of transvestites is rather similar to that of homosexuals. The transvestite is asked in the experimental laboratory to put on the pieces of feminine wear which he usually enjoys; after putting on each piece electric shocks are given, and conversely shock is stopped whenever he removes a female piece of clothing. Treatment of transvestism is similar in many ways, as far as success is concerned, to alcoholism and homosexuality; no new or different problems arise.

As a case history to illustrate the application of aversion therapy I have chosen a case of fetishism originally published by

Dr M. J. Raymond from St George's Hospital in London. The patient was a married man aged thirty-three who had been considered for a prefrontal leucotomy operation after he had attacked a perambulator. This was the twelfth such attack known to the police, and because of the previous incidents they were taking a serious view of his actions in following a woman with a perambulator and smearing it with oil. The patient said he had had impulses to damage perambulators and handbags since about the age of ten, and that although the police knew of only twelve perambulator attacks, the number of times he had so indulged was legion. He had sometimes made several attacks in one day, but he estimated an average of two or three attacks a week, fairly consistently. As regards handbags, he was usually satisfied if he could scratch them with a thumb nail, and as this could be unobtrusively done, handbags had only led him once into trouble with the police!

He had received many hours of psychoanalytic treatment, without success. He traced his abnormality back to two incidents in his childhood. On one occasion he had been taken to a park to sail his boat and had been impressed by the feminine consternation manifest when he struck the keel of his boat against a passing perambulator. The second occasion was when he became sexually aroused in the presence of his sister's handbag. Psychoanalysts had led him to see the significance of these events and to understand them: perambulators and handbags were for him 'symbolic sexual containers'. Nevertheless, the attacks continued. He had masturbated with fantasies of prams and handbags from the age of ten, and intercourse later on was only possible with the aid of fantasies of handbags and prams.

The therapist explained to the patient that the aim of treatment was to alter his attitude to handbags and perambulators by teaching him to associate them with an unpleasant sensation instead of with a pleasurable erotic sensation. The patient was very sceptical about the treatment but agreed to participate. The therapist obtained a collection of handbags, perambulators and coloured illustrations and showed these to the patient after he had received an injection of apomorphine, and just before nausea was produced. Treatment continued for about three weeks, with interruptions, and the patient found he was able to have intercourse with his wife without the use of the old fantasies; he also lost all desire to have any dealings with handbags and perambulators. A booster course of treatment was given after six months although there does not seem to have been a relapse in any case, and nineteen months after he had first had aversion therapy he was still doing well when contacted. He has not been in any trouble with the police, has a more responsible job and has improved in many other ways. The treatment had no undesirable after-effects.

The second case may illustrate the application of aversion therapy to a case of obesity. The patient was a twenty-six-year-old woman who weighed fifteen stone on admission; she had been taking amphetamine periodically for some six years, ostensibly to help her to reduce weight. She was treated initially by withdrawal of amphetamine and by psychotherapy. She did quite well in a strongly supported therapeutic relationship and her weight fell to twelve stone. However, when the therapist left the hospital, and social rehabilitation was attempted, the patient relapsed immediately. She reverted to taking amphetamine and over-eating until her weight went up to sixteen stone. The patient's conscious need remained that of losing weight and of being slim and attractive. The therapists, Drs V. Meyer and A. H. Crisp, agreed that if this could be achieved her general interpersonal relationships might improve; otherwise she was considered practically untreatable except by compulsory detention.

Treatment consisted of putting the patient on a basic 1,000 calorie diet and placing her in an isolation room containing a one-way screen. Her weight chart was placed on the wall with a photograph of an obese subject at the level of the upper weight range and a slim, attractive subject at the level of the therapeutically desired weight level (ten stone). A transformer, designed to give electric shocks of varying voltages, was placed outside the room. Two electrodes were attached to the patient's left arm. The specific procedure for treatment was as follows. The 'temptation food' – some kind of food for which the patient had most craving – was displayed for increasing periods of time in the room. Any approach by the patient towards this food was punished by shock to prevent eating, the strength of the shock being set at an uncomfortable level for the patient. The patient was never shocked while eating her prescribed diet.

This treatment lasted for about six weeks. In the first treatment session the patient required five shocks; during about thirty subsequent sessions she frequently made no approach to the 'temptation food' at all; on the five occasions when she did, she immediately received further shocks which were always stopped when she stopped her approach to the food. From the time she ceased to make any form of approach behaviour towards the 'temptation food' the possibility of receiving immediate shock was progressively reduced; first by disconnecting plugs, then by removing the electrodes on the patient's arm, and finally by removing all the electrical appliances from the room. The patient was also told that she would not be constantly observed in the presence of the 'temptation food'. Eventually she was given increasing social and dietary freedom under part observation. Her weight was plotted daily.

During the six weeks of treatment the patient lost weight (from 205 to 185 lbs). During the next six months she continued to lose weight steadily. At the time of discharge her weight had been constant for three months at between 113 and 120 lbs. Following treatment she had persisted with the low calorie diet and had become reluctant to eat even this at times. Twenty months after treatment she weighed 133 lbs and said that her weight had not fluctuated greatly.

Before closing this chapter we must mention one theoretical difficulty that attaches to the explanation of aversion therapy. It is possible, as we have seen, to consider it as a simple case of Pavlovian conditioning, but it is also possible to look upon it in a rather different light. It is customary in psychology to distinguish between two rather different kinds of conditioning, the one called Pavlovian or classical, the other instrumental or operant. The distinction may be made clear by recounting rather similar experiments conducted by Pavlov and the Russian physiologist Bechterev, Pavlov's great rival at the time of the First World War. In one of Pavlov's experiments he would use a set of electrodes firmly attached to the foot of a dog; shock through these electrodes to the dog's foot would be the unconditioned stimulus, leading to the response of lifting the leg and flexing the knee. The conditioned stimulus was a bell. After a while the dog responded with flexing the knee and lifting the leg to the sound of the bell, even though no shock was given. It is important to realise that the shock did not cease when the animal lifted his leg but continued irrespective of the dog's movement until the preordained duration of shock had elapsed. In other words the dog did not gain anything by lifting his leg; it was simply a natural reflex which could later be evoked by the conditioned stimulus.

Bechterev's experiment was subtly different. Here the dog would stand with his foot on a metal grid which could be electrified. The conditioned stimulus was a bell again, and shortly after the bell had sounded, the grid would be electrified, and the dog would lift his foot. However in this case lifting the foot would end the shock; in other words the conditioned response was instrumental in producing an effect. This is the origin of the term 'instrumental conditioning'; more recently B. F. Skinner, the Harvard behaviourist psychologist, has suggested the term 'operant conditioning' as a synonym for 'instrumental conditioning'. The two methods of conditioning show many dissimilarities as well as similarities, and it is usually assumed nowadays that they define two rather different types of learning. Pavlovian or classical conditioning seems more closely related to the learning of emotional responses, whereas instrumental or operant conditioning is more closely related to the learning of behaviour patterns.

We have presented aversion therapy as a kind of Pavlovian conditioning; in other words, we have assumed that the particular reaction that is being conditioned is a feeling of fear/anxiety, and that it is this feeling which later on determines the avoidance behaviour demonstrated by the patient. However, we might look upon the whole course of conditioning rather from the operant, B. F. Skinner point of view, and regard it as a case of instrumental conditioning. Moving away from the alcohol or the fellow homosexual or the fetishistic objects is instrumental in avoiding punishment, and therefore continues as the preferred type of behaviour. There are many theoretical problems raised by this distinction between classical and instrumental conditioning but they need not concern us here unduly. The distinction is introduced mainly for the sake of completeness, but also because it is very relevant to the next type of treatment which we shall consider, namely the so-called token economy. This is almost certainly more closely related to the instrumental type of conditioning, although we cannot rule out entirely the presence of elements of classical conditioning as well. It has always proved very difficult to mark a clear distinction between the two, even in the laboratory, but fortunately from the point of view of our description here we need not be too concerned with refinements of this type.

Token economies

The term 'token economy' was introduced into psychological parlance by Teodoro Ayllon and Nathan Azrin, then of the Anna State Hospital in Georgia, USA. The term refers to a method of treatment which combines two major ideas, both of which have good psychological backing. The first one we have already encountered; it asserts that conditioning is most effective when the interval between conditioned and unconditioned stimulus is very short. The other idea is that punishment can have such variable consequences that it is often of no use in modifying human conduct (or animal conduct for that matter). We have already given an example of the odd effects of punishment in connection with the shuttlebox experiment in which dogs were conditioned to jump over the fence separating the two parts of the room; it will be remembered that once they had been conditioned, they continued their behaviour even though the current was switched in such a way that they received a shock on jumping into the previously safe chamber. In other words, their habits of jumping became stronger rather than weaker for being punished. In a similar way it has often been found that birching juvenile delinquents makes them if anything even more set in their ways, rather than persuading them of the undesirability of continuing their mugging, vandalism and criminality in general.

Some psychologists have taken this too far and allege that all punishment is not only vile but counter-productive. This is clearly untrue, and the psychological literature is full of studies which demonstrate the absurdity of this proposition. What can be said, however, is that the use of punishment is nothing like as simple and straightforward as the layman imagines; punishing a person for indulging in a certain course of activity may suppress that activity while the threat of punishment is present, but it does not abolish it, and once the threat is removed the same course of action will again be followed. For permanent rehabilitation punishment may not be a suitable method of treatment, and it may be better to look for a method using rewards rather than punishments. Following Professor Skinner it has become the usual practice to refer to rewards and punishments in a proper conditioning situation as positive and negative reinforcements. The terms are clumsy, but they do go beyond reward and punishment in suggesting certain experimental parameters, such as immediacy or contingency of conditioned and unconditioned stimulus: this makes them more precise and useful. For this reason they will be used in our discussion.

In a proper token economy we start out with a kind of contract between the therapist and the patient. We shall continue to use these terms although in the case of behaviour modification with criminals the term 'patient' may strike the observer as odd, and the term 'therapist' as inappropriate. This contract specifies clearly the types of behaviour which the therapist and/or the patient may wish to see changed, and it also specifies that on any occasion when the preferred behaviour is manifested by the patient a token will be given to him by the therapist or his representative which the patient can then exchange later on for any of a given range of 'goodies'. These rewards vary widely in nature but may be cigarettes, sweets, or any other suitable reward.

Let us assume that our setting is a rather unruly classroom, and that the teacher wishes to induce more orderly behaviour in his pupils. In the ordinary way he would probably try punishment, but this is of doubtful value; it often does not work, and in any case it may produce a highly undesirable hostility towards the teacher on the part of the pupils. The alternative would be to introduce a token economy, in which the teacher lays down specific aspects of the behaviour which he wants members of the class to manifest, and also the numbers of tokens which will be given to pupils who demonstrate this kind of behaviour. There are of course practical difficulties in observing pupils constantly, administering the tokens, and finally exchanging them for the requisite range of 'goodies'. However, these difficulties can be overcome, at least in experimental sessions, and it has been shown often enough that the method is extremely powerful and useful. Not only does it work like a charm with the most obstructive sets of pupils, it also produces a positive relationship between teacher and children which is highly desirable and can be exploited in many different ways. The situation can of course get out of hand, until it is not very clear who is conditioning whom. In one experiment the psychologist decided to introduce a token economy in the morning, but leave the afternoon class in its original form, in order to retain a baseline against which to measure the changes produced by the token economy. The children enjoyed the token economy version so much that they wanted it introduced in the afternoon also; to this end they began to misbehave so atrociously in the afternoon that the teacher had to give way and introduce a token economy in the afternoon as well! The whole episode recalls the famous cartoon in which the experimental rat proudly explains to his country cousin: 'I really have my psychologist conditioned properly now; whenever I press a lever he drops a pellet of food into my hopper!'

While the scientific principles on which the token economy is based may be new, the method itself certainly is not. It was originally invented by a British penologist, Alexander Maconochie, who introduced his very original 'mark system of discipline' in Norfold Island, one of the most cruel and soul-destroying of all convict settlements which the English Government instituted in Australia. Maconochie was appointed superintendent of Norfold Island in 1840; he found conditions there corresponding exactly to those described in a famous sentence by the Reverend Sidney Smith, who in 1822 declared that the prison should be 'a place of punishment from which men recoiled with horror − a place of real suffering, painful to the memory, terrible to the imagination . . . A place of sorrow and wailing, which could be entered with horror and left with earnest resolution never to return to such misery; with that deep impression, in short, of the evil which breaks out into perpetual warning and exhortation to others.' Maconochie's view was very different. 'I think that time sentences are the root of very nearly all the demoralization which exists in prison. A man under a time sentence thinks only how he is to cheat that time, and while it away; he hates labour, because he has no interest in it whatever, and he has no desire to please the officers under whom he is placed, because they cannot serve him essentially; they cannot in any way promote his liberation . . . Now these . . . evils would be remedied by introducing the system of task sentences.'

Maconochie in other words proposed the substitution of the task rather than the time sentence; instead of being sentenced to imprisonment for a period of time, the offender should be sentenced to be imprisoned until he had performed a specified quantity of labour. To specify and quantify this amount of labour is of course difficult; Maconochie suggested that the prisoner should be ordered to earn by labour and other forms of good conduct a fixed number of 'marks of commendation', and that his period of detention should end only when he had done so. On first entering the prison, the offender would suffer a short period of restraint and deprivation; this would shortly be followed by a second stage during which he could earn privileges, as well as shelter and food, by the earnings from his labour and good conduct. Purchases could be made by computing the value of the goods in 'marks', then setting them off against the 'marks' earned by the prisoner. The performance of allotted tasks would thus enable him to earn a daily tally of marks, for example, ten marks, but by frugal living, constant industry beyond the allotted task, and exemplary behaviour and demeanour, he could add to the daily tally. Disciplinary offences would not be punished by the customary prison methods of violence, deprivation, or enforced labour, but by fines expressed in marks, and by the withdrawal of privileges.

As a third stage, prisoners were permitted to join with other prisoners and engage in the performance of joint work projects in which the misconduct of one member was punished by loss of marks by the whole group.

> As a prisoner progressed through the system, the restraints upon him should be lessened, and the final period of his detention should resemble as much as possible the conditions likely to be encountered on release, the express purpose of this stage being to prepare him for the release which the whole system was devised to enable him to achieve by his own efforts. The fundamental principle was: nothing for nothing; everything must be earned. Throughout the period of detention anything that tended to degrade the prisoner, or to deprive him of the character 'social being' should be avoided. Brutal punishment such as the use of leg irons, the wearing of chains, 'spread eagling', the gag and the lash, should not be used.

Maconochie, in spite of all sorts of official opposition from the Home Office, carried these ideas into effect; I have described this in some detail in my book *Psychology is about People* and will not do so again here. The outcome of the experiment, insofar as it can be evaluated, seems to be very favourable to Maconochie's ideas; against the background of official policy at the time, the success of his particular system of token economy seems almost miraculous.

Token economies very similar to those used by Alexander Maconochie 135 years ago have been experimented with in recent years, particularly in the United States. Most work has been done with deteriorated schizophrenics, who receive tokens for such activities as getting up on their own, making their bed, going to have their meals on time, eating their meals by themselves, working in the laundry or at some other job, and performing a variety of acts which restore them to a semblance of normal life. Occasionally in this way patients have been improved so much that they could be let out into the community at large, but on the whole it is probable that they are not *cured* by these methods but rather that the methods of the token economy counteract the ill effects of hospital life, where being in a very restricted environment and being so institutionalized for a large number of years produces very undesirable effects on behaviour which may be even worse than the actual disease which originally sent the patient into hospital.

An example may make it clear what I have in mind. You want to train a young puppy to obey commands. You throw a ball, and he runs after it and takes it in his mouth. You order him to come back to you, but he pays no attention and just rushes around wildly. You keep calling, and he doesn't come. Finally he does condescend to come to you. Normally an owner would get annoyed at the constant disobedience and perhaps beat the dog; however this would be quite counter-productive because the conditioning paradigm would now read, for the dog: 'Be good - come - get beaten!' This means that the next time he would be even less likely to come. What the owner should do would be to reward (provide positive reinforcement for) the little segment of obedient behaviour produced by the dog; in this way the dog's conditioning will read: 'Get called – come – get rewarded.' Consequently the next time he is called he will be more likely to come, and by constant reinforcement the owner will finally get to the point where the dog is trained.

In the typical mental hospital, nurses pay attention to the patient when he is unruly, obstreperous, or generally misbehaves;

in other words he is rewarded (by having attention paid to him) for undesirable behaviours, and in this way the undesirable behaviours are stamped in, and desirable behaviours stamped out! If this is continued over a period of twenty or thirty years, no wonder the patient, whatever the stage of his illness, behaves in an outrageous manner. This problem can only be counteracted by something of the nature of a token economy, a method of psychological management which does exactly the opposite and reinforces good, desirable behaviour instead of reinforcing bad, undesirable behaviour.

Unfortunately what is true of the hospital, or of the amateur training his dog, is also true of the way many people bring up children. Mother is usually too busy to pay attention to the children when they are being good; she only starts paying attention when they play up. In other words, their bad behaviour is rewarded by having mother pay attention whereas good behaviour is not rewarded because mother is too busy to pay attention! In this way mother stamps in bad behaviour and eliminates good behaviour; she then wonders why her children are not the little angels the textbooks on child upbringing promised her! The principles of positive and negative reinforcement may be very simple, so simple in fact that most people will regard them as nothing but common sense; nevertheless, in every day life we constantly behave as if we had never heard of these principles and didn't believe in them – in fact we usually act in such a way as to produce the opposite effects to those we would like to produce.

Token economies have been used in many different connections, as with deteriorated schizophrenics, with criminals, and also in marriages that are in danger of breaking down. Married partners often do not realise that the basis of a good marriage is a mutual reinforcement pattern – I reinforce you by doing what you want, if you reinforce me by doing what I want. In many marriages the partners are too tongue-tied to be able to tell each other what they want, and consequently fail to reinforce each other positively. The therapist can introduce a token economy, by getting each partner to write down in detail the behaviours which he wishes his or her partner to show; for each demonstration of such behaviours the partner is then given a number of tokens. These tokens can then be used to 'buy' the kind of behaviour that partner wants. The method is clumsy, and sounds as if it were a bad joke, but for people who are rather dull and unable to express their feelings it has possibilities; several studies show that it works very well in practice, with certain people.

The methods of instrumental or operant conditioning, as applied to the treatment of mental disorders, criminality, classroom unrest, marriage upsets, etc., have been used on a much larger scale than has been indicated in this chapter. Skinner and his followers have in fact extrapolated the results of laboratory experiments with rats and pigeons not only to the treatment of mental abnormalities and criminal behaviour but to the very organization of society, to religion and to the whole question of 'freedom and dignity'. This extrapolation, based upon a single general law, namely that of 'effect', or positive and negative reinforcement, is so speculative and absurd that nothing further will be said here about it. Insofar as there are empirical studies using instrumental conditioning along Skinnerian lines, they have been concerned with autistic children, schizophrenic patients, and other groups which are not relevant to a book on neurosis. As far as the treatment of neurotic patients is concerned, there has been very little application of Skinnerian principles.

Skinnerian behaviourism has become a 'school', in the same way as Freudianism did many years earlier. Skinnerians concentrate exclusively on a very small area of psychology, disregard the great mass of empirical data not reduceable to explanation in terms of positive and negative reinforcement, and proselytize in the manner of religious prophets; in all this they very much resemble members of the Freudian school. Their methods are certainly impressive in the results achieved under certain very unusual circumstances. Behaviour therapists are aware of the power of these methods but would usually deny their applicability to the wide range of neurotic disorders which mostly claim their attention. The term 'behaviour modification' has sometimes been used to distinguish the methods of instrumental or operant conditioning from other types of behaviour therapy, although this usage is by no means universal; some people use the terms behaviour therapy and behaviour modification as almost synonymous. There may be an advantage in making this distinction, and if we do so it must be said that, as far as the treatment of neurotic disorders is concerned, Pavlovian conditioning and behaviour therapy have proved vastly more useful than behaviour modification and the principles of instrumental or operant conditioning.

An example may illustrate the use of the principles of instrumental conditioning in cases where they may be properly applied. The case is that of a paranoid woman suffering from ideas of persecution. She was convinced that the communists were after her and wanted to kill her and rob her of all her money. She discharged herself from a hospital in England and flew to the United States, convinced that communists were less likely to be found there. However, when she left the plane she encountered a Chinese-looking gentleman and this convinced her that she had been wrong; she immediately flew back and returned to the mental hospital from which she had discharged herself. Treatment along Skinnerian lines was begun by having her sit opposite to the psychologist, who had in front of him a bell push. The patient was wearing earphones and whenever she started talking about her paranoid ideas, the psychologist would push the button and white noise would be relayed over the earphones until she changed the subject. After a few sessions of this method of operant conditioning she ceased to talk about her ideas, and this habit spread to the ward and elsewhere. To make sure that the method of treatment was responsible for this change, rather than some kind of spontaneous remission, the psychologist now reversed the process and positively reinforced talk about her paranoid ideas. This was successful in bringing them back in full flood, and during the next few weeks the psychologist reversed the process several times at will until he was finally convinced that the method was working. The final few sessions removed the paranoid ideas from her talking repertoire, and follow-up showed that for all practical purposes she was 'cured', and could go out into the world again and return to her family. The term 'cure' is put in quotation marks because it is perhaps unlikely that the ideas themselves were entirely eliminated by this process. It was only the act of talking about them which originally led to her being sent to the hospital, and her success in eliminating this habit of giving voice to her ideas made it possible for her to live a reasonably ordinary life again. Note however that this was a psychotic, not a neurotic patient; neurotic symptoms are more resistant to instrumental conditioning, and little in the way of success has been reported in the literature as far as treatment of neuroses by Skinnerian methods is concerned.

6 Neurosis and Society

The effects of therapy

So far in this book we have considered psychological theories
and quoted individual case studies to illustrate the principles of
treatment based upon these theories. The fact that these case
studies had a more or less satisfactory outcome does not prove the
correctness of the theories or the usefulness of the methods of
treatment, unfortunately. What is required, of course, is a series
of clinical trials, in which the improvement shown by patients
treated by the methods under examination is compared with that
observed in patients receiving no treatment at all, receiving other
types of treatment, and receiving placebo or 'dummy' treatment.
Why are these complications necessary?

The first and most important fact about neuroses is that they
are *self-limiting*; in other words, sufferers tend to get better
without any form of psychiatric or medical treatment. This, as
we have already seen, is called *spontaneous remission*, although the
suggestion contained in this phrase that remission is really spontaneous, in the sense of being uncaused, is certainly erroneous.
Remission occurs over time, but it must be presumed that it is
events occurring during that time which determine the final outcome. We have already discussed some possible causes of spontaneous remission, such as extinction due to the repeated unreinforced presentation of the conditioned stimulus. This would constitute a kind of unplanned and accidental application of desensitization or flooding, working much less well than a properly
planned and executed application of these methods, and always
open to the possibility of disaster, but nevertheless therapeutic for
the most part. Another possibility is that while sufferers may not
approach the psychiatrist for help, they may seek such help from
priests, from friends, from quacks, or in other ways; there is
much evidence to show that psychiatrists and psychologists are
much less frequently consulted than other sources of help, such as

those named. Their ministrations also are likely to be unplanned and unscientific, but they may, and no doubt often do, provide unsystematic but in the long run effective desensitization for the troubled sufferer. Figure 11 shows the percentage improvement of seriously ill neurotic patients over the years when no psychiatric treatment is administered.

The extent of spontaneous remission is not always realized, but the consensus of a large number of varied studies may be summed up by saying that on the whole some two out of three neurotics, suffering from fairly serious to very serious disorders, improve greatly or recover completely over a period of two years or so when not receiving any psychiatric treatment. This is a high proportion, and must always be borne in mind when assessing the effects of any method of therapy. If people get better by themselves, without treatment, then clearly a particular method of treatment must do better than that; it would not be sufficient to point to a recovery rate of two out of three and claim that this proved the efficacy of the treatment! In the past all sorts of treatments, many quite grotesque and useless, such as cold baths, hot showers, or the extraction of all one's teeth in order to eliminate septic foci, have been claimed to be successful, with a proud showing of a two-thirds rate of recovery after two years. Such a rate of improvement simply shows the method up as completely useless. Thus a 'control group' not receiving treatment should always be included in the design of a study to determine the relative usefulness of a particular therapy; without it we may simply be reaping the benefits of spontaneous recovery.

The use of such a group of patients receiving no treatment is particularly important because while the two out of three figure for spontaneous recovery is an accurate enough estimate overall, there is good evidence to show that different types of neurotic disorder recover at different rates. Thus specific phobias and obsessive-compulsive disorders are particularly slow to recover, and very frequently may not recover at all without treatment; it is for this reason that most of our examples have been chosen from these groups. Personality disorders and psychopaths are in the same category of patients showing little spontaneous remission; so are alcoholics and homosexuals. Patients suffering from anxiety conditions generally recover most quickly, and it is with them, of course, that psychotherapists have claimed their greatest

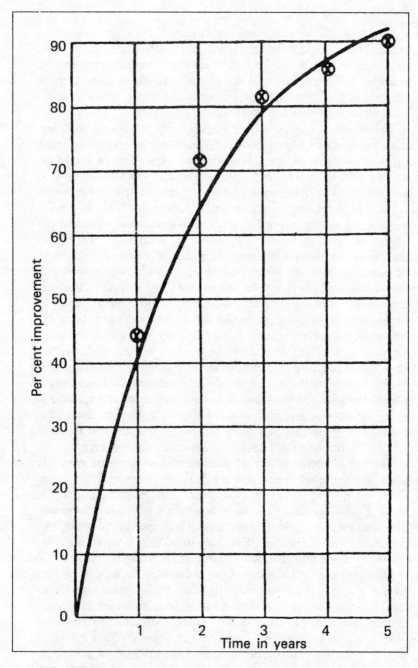

FIGURE 11
Improvement of seriously ill neurotic patients receiving
no psychiatric treatment. (Sample: 500 patients.)

successes. For any scientific assessment of the effectiveness of a given type of therapy, therefore, it is not sufficient to compare results with an overall figure of two out of three for spontaneous remission; a no-treatment group is required which must be similar in make-up to the treatment group, in order to equalize differences in remission rate due to differences in symptomatology.

The provision of such a control group obviously raises all sorts of ethical problems – are we justified in withholding treatment from patients for purely scientific purposes? The problem is intricate, but let me here simply state briefly my answer to this objection. No method of treatment should be used routinely unless and until it has been shown to work; withholding treatment the effectiveness of which is in doubt, and which may in fact have deleterious consequences for the patient, can hardly be unethical.[1] Exactly the reverse is true. Electroshock treatment is very widely given in mental hospitals, yet there has never been a proper study of its effectiveness, as compared with matched control groups! The treatment is cruel, violent, and undoubtedly may have serious side-effects and after-effects. Can we justify such methods of treatment without proof of their effectiveness? Many psychiatrists have answered this question in the negative, and the so-called anti-psychiatry lobby has come out strongly against the use of electroshock treatment, and of brain surgery of the leucotomy type, for which also evidence is pitifully meagre.[2]

---

[1] Medical and ethical objections to the use of control trials are not of course only voiced in connection with psychiatric treatment. A good example comes from the introduction of intensive coronary care units; a clinical test of the effectiveness of these units was carried out against considerable medical opposition, the argument being that it was unethical to withhold this treatment from the control group, who were treated in their homes. As it happened, the results of the trial were negative – patients treated at home did slightly better than those treated in the coronary care units. One should never confuse an apparently good idea with an idea which has actually been tried out and found successful; this differentiation is natural to scientists, but medical men and laymen often confuse the two. It is not unethical to withhold treatment for the effectiveness of which there does not exist any sound scientific evidence.

[2] It should not be imagined that electroshock treatment and other physical psychiatric methods are unusual in medical practice as being both dangerous and of doubtful use. Tonsillectomy is more dangerous than ECT (one in every thousand children who have their tonsils removed is killed by the operation, and sixteen are made seriously ill; this should be compared with a fatality figure of 1 in 50,000 due to a single administration of ECT.) Removing the tonsils also quadruples the risk of catching bulbar polio and triples the risk of Hodgkins disease (a form of cancer usually fatal). The indications for

The problem is made easier in the case of psychotherapy by the fact that many people who are judged likely to benefit from the treatment, and for whom it is recommended by psychotherapists, either cannot receive it at all, or receive it only after a long wait because of the scarcity of psychotherapists and of financial resources. It would be easy to make up a control group of such people who in any case would not receive psychotherapy during the experimental period. As a recompense, they might then be admitted to psychotherapy immediately afterwards, thus benefiting on the whole from the arrangement. It is an interesting sidelight on spontaneous remission that of the patients placed upon a waiting list, a fair proportion say they no longer require treatment when called to the hospital after six months or so.

Why do we need a placebo or 'dummy treatment' group? The answer is simply this. It is well known that suggestibility plays a large part in mental healing. Any treatment, however absurd, will benefit from this suggestibility on the part of the patient, at least in the short run. Since we are interested in the specific effects of those aspects of the treatment which we are intending to test, we must have a measure of the influence of suggestibility, in order to be able to subtract this from the observed effectiveness of our own therapy. Only what remains is then a genuine effect, attributable specifically to our treatment. Even physical symptoms, like pain, have been shown to be strongly influenced by suggestion; dummy tablets containing nothing but flour and sugar have often been shown to be almost as effective in reducing physical pain as morphine and aspirin. Thus we must guard against this effect very carefully. Here again, of course, ethical considerations come in to obscure the picture, and the same answers may be given as in the case of simple no-treatment control groups.

---

tonsillectomy are quite unclear and agreement among doctors in individual cases is notable for its absence; unreliability here is at least as great as it is in the case of psychiatric diagnosis!

Readers who feel that perhaps I have been too hard on the lack of evidence for the effectiveness of ECT may like to ponder the following (factual and documented) story. After an ECT machine had been installed in a British mental hospital and used for six months, it was discovered that through a wiring fault the machine was not delivering any current. The doctors using it had not noticed that it was not functioning, nor had they noticed any difference in the effects of the treatment on their patients from that expected from a properly functioning machine. The facts speak for themselves.

Ideally we would want to have more than one treatment group, in order to compare the specific effects, say, of psychotherapy and behaviour therapy, and of course the number of groups could be enlarged endlessly to accommodate the many different types of behaviour therapy and psychotherapy. But for a beginning one would be quite content to have a single study which fulfilled these major requirements, as well as one or two minor ones. Thus each type of therapy would have to be practised on different patients by more than one exponent of the different types of therapy in question. Obviously, if Dr Smith, using the methods of behaviour therapy, does better than Dr Jones, using the methods of psychotherapy, this might indicate that behaviour therapy was better than psychotherapy: it might also show, instead, that Dr Smith was a better therapist than Dr Jones, irrespective of the method of treatment! We should also require a good, reliable and objective measure of the effectiveness of therapy, and this is very difficult to provide. Perhaps the judgment of improvement made by a third party, ignorant of the method of treatment applied, might be acceptable, together with certain objective physiological and behavioural criteria. This in itself is an intricate issue on which many pages could be written.

How do methods of treatment in psychiatry stand up to these criteria? The answer is a melancholy one. We have already noted that physical methods, such as electroshock and leucotomy, lack proper support in well-controlled clinical investigations; this is a major scandal which fully justifies the criticisms made by the antipsychiatry school of psychiatrists. But the position is no better as far as psychotherapy is concerned; there is no single study which fulfils the requirements, elementary as they are, suggested above. What we have is a set of about a hundred studies noting the effectiveness of psychotherapy, or of psychoanalysis, on poorly designated samples, lacking follow-ups, and relying entirely on the final judgment of the therapist himself (prejudiced as he may be in favour of his own effectiveness). Occasionally a rather inadequate control group is provided, but usually the principles of selection are different for this group than for the experimental group. Placebo treatments are practically never given. This is a sorry list of failures; what is the overall outcome of therapy so assessed? Lo and behold, it just about equals the magic figure of two out of three recovered or much improved! In other words, the existing evidence, poor as it is, suggests that psychotherapy has on the whole no influence at all – the patients would have got better just as quickly, and just as markedly, had they never seen a psychotherapist. The voluminous literature has been carefully surveyed by Dr S. Rachman, in his book on *The Effects of Psychotherapy*. He concludes that there is no proper evidence in favour of the effectiveness of psychotherapy. This conclusion may have to be qualified by noting that there is some evidence that psychotherapy may have harmful effects; some writers have shown that the effects of psychotherapy depend greatly on the personality of the therapist, with some (impersonal, cold, non-supportive) making the neurotic patient worse, and others (warm, supportive, empathic) making him better. It is possible that these contrasting effects may balance out, leaving psychotherapy as neither harmful nor helpful on the whole. Needless to say, this conclusion also is not based on adequate evidence. All that we are entitled to say is that *no evidence exists on which a positive verdict in favour of the effectiveness of psychotherapy or psychoanalysis could be pronounced*; in view of the long-continued failure to provide such evidence some psychologists and psychiatrists have concluded that the answer probably is simply that these methods in fact have no effect. This may very well be so, but it is difficult to prove a negative. What we may perhaps say is that, if psychotherapy has any effect, it must be small and evanescent on the whole, unless indeed good and bad effects balance out. Either way, to train whole generations of psychiatrists in this 'art', and to submit many thousands of sufferers from neurotic illness to these doubtfully efficacious methods, seems unrealistic and undesirable.

We have noted already the absence of follow-ups in most of these investigations; this is a crucial point. Even if the immediate effects of psychotherapy could be shown to be better than those of no treatment, or of placebo treatment, such effects might be short-lived. Studies have been done to show that the immediate outcome of psychiatric treatment and the long-term outcome are poorly correlated; patients often show an up-and-down effect in their symptoms which frequently leads to the termination of treatment when the patient is at the top of his wave, giving the illusory impression of success for the treatment. This is the so-called 'hello – goodbye' effect. After termination of treatment the patient often slumps back into his neurosis, only to go and seek out another doctor who repeats the 'hello – goodbye' effect. Long-term follow-up studies are required to give a proper estimate of the true effects of treatment. Such studies as have been done do not assuage our uneasiness in this respect.

Investigation into the effects of psychotherapy, and particularly of psychoanalysis, is handicapped most by the long duration of these therapies. An average of four years is probably not unrealistic where psychoanalysis is concerned, and psychotherapy is also usually fairly prolonged, although seldom quite as much. Analyses of twenty years' duration, or even more, are not unknown; clearly so much happens to the neurotic during such long periods of time that to apportion responsibility between treatment and the ordinary events of his life becomes very difficult. Psychoanalysts themselves have often admitted that there seems to be little correspondence between events in the analytic treatment session, and the ups and downs of the patient's emotional life; such correspondence is absolutely necessary if the theory is to retain any credibility whatever. No studies exist to demonstrate correspondence of this kind. With very short-term therapies, like most of the methods of behaviour therapy, it is much easier to establish causal links and demonstrate effectiveness; if in a patient who has been ill for twenty or more years, and has undergone many different types of therapy, both psychotherapy and physical therapy, without success, desensitization or flooding produce startling and permanent effects within a period of a few weeks, or months at the most, then we can be fairly confident that this is not the effect of placebos, nor a simple temporary upswing, nor spontaneous remission – not if the treatment is efficacious in many subsequent cases also.

The finding that psychotherapy and psychoanalysis are so strangely ineffective is surprising in many ways. Treatments so widely used, so extravagantly praised and advertised, and so expensive in time and money would normally be expected to have some observable effect, other than to make the patient 'a better person' while leaving his symptoms unaffected. Perhaps there is more than an analogy with the ancient practice of bleeding patients, and setting leeches on them. This too was totally ineffective, and probably did more harm than good, but it continued over many centuries as the sovereign remedy for all sorts of physical and mental ills.

Surprise at the ineffectiveness of psychoanalysis comes from another quarter, too. Patients for this type of treatment are carefully selected by the analyst; they tend to be white, wealthy, youngish, well educated, bright, and with some measure of 'ego strength', meaning that they are not badly ill. In other words, it is precisely those patients who are selected for psychotherapy who are most likely to recover spontaneously: surely they should do better than a random group of neurotics, including the dull, the coloured, the old, the poorly educated, and the sufferers with weak egos, who receive no treatment at all! (Something like two-thirds of all applicants for psychoanalytic treatment are refused, so this gives some idea of the amount of selection practised.) The fact that no such differences in outcome have been demonstrated makes it all the more likely that in fact the methods of treatment here considered have little or no effect on the neurotic disorders the patients complain about.

What do psychoanalysts reply to these charges? In the first place, as already noted, analysts have retreated from the position held at the heyday of Freudian supremacy in psychiatry, when they claimed that psychoanalysis was the only method which cured neurotic patients, and that it did so more or less as a matter of course. (I have many statements to this effect in my files.) Nowadays claims are much more modest; it is said that psychoanalysis makes the patient more able to cope with his symptoms, or makes him a better person in some unspecified way; claims for proper cures are conspicuously missing. This is sometimes accompanied by a denial of the possibility of cures altogether. These are modest claims, impossible to test because they are so vague as to be meaningless.

Others claim that the tests so far done are unfair. Good effects are claimed when the right therapist meets the right patient; in other words, there is no general method, applicable to all neurotics, nor a good therapist, able to treat all patients, but a specific combination of doctor and patient where everything clicks into place and a miraculous cure is produced. This is possible, but as a claim it is untestable; all successes could be claimed as favouring the hypothesis, all failures could be shrugged off as simply instances of bad fit, thus also favouring the hypothesis.

Unless the 'fit' can be specified prior to treatment (and no one has suggested how this can be done) this hypothesis won't do; it is untestable, and hence beyond science. It is true that type of personality and method of treatment interact, in a predictable fashion, as we shall see, but this applies to behavioural methods, and nothing comparable has been demonstrated in relation to psychotherapy.

It is possible that a clue to the mystery of discovering the type of person who is likely to benefit from psychotherapy has been supplied by Dr H.B.M. Murphy, of the Hôpital du Sacré-Coeur in Montreal. He used two groups of neurotic patients; half were given psychotherapy, the other half no psychiatric treatment. As expected, this made no difference to recovery; both groups did equally well. However, it proved possible to select out a group of patients who clearly benefited from psychotherapy and did much better when given this treatment than when not given it. These patients showed two characteristics in combination. In the first place, they were introverted; extraverts did not show any differences due to treatment. In the second place, they had some 'gumption' – they had no recent absence from work, they were able to voice anger at frustration, they had not recently taken psychotropic drugs, and they found life difficult but manageable. As Dr Murphy says,

> It would appear that it is the underlying personality rather than the current ailment which determines whether specialist care is needed in the neuroses. The neurotic patients in our sample who most benefited from psychiatric treatment and did least well without it were introverts who had always thought themselves to be rather unhealthy but who had refused to say that life was becoming too much for them and had avoided the easy solutions of taking time off from work or using drugs. They were people who seemed able to converse easily and consult others regarding their own problems, so that they probably did not appear so introverted to others, and they could apparently handle frustrations without either repressing their irritation or losing self-control.

Why do such apparently competent persons need psychotherapy? Murphy answers that it may be their very competence that has trapped them.

They would seem likely to have got into the habit of tackling their problems in a particular fashion, but have exhausted themselves in fruitlessly applying that method to their present situation. The average psychiatrist would probe deeply enough to recognize this and to suggest a new method of self-aid.

This study is in urgent need of replication, and this particular hypothesis is at present little more than guess-work. However, should replication prove successful, then we might say that for one small group of neurotics, amounting to something like 15 per cent of all sufferers who come for treatment, psychotherapy may have some use. (Behaviour therapy, of course, might be even better.)

We must next turn to behaviour therapy and ask the same question: does behaviour therapy work? In saying that the answer must be that it does, I would not wish to be understood as saying that the proof for this assertion is overwhelmingly strong and definitive. Considering the complexity of the issues involved, and the difficulty of mounting a proper study of therapeutic effectiveness, general statements must inevitably be suspect. More circumscribed statements, however, can be made, such as that methods of response prevention are highly successful in cases of obsessive-compulsive disorder, or that methods of desensitization are very successful in cases of phobic fears or general anxieties. Follow-up studies have been done, but inevitably these only cover limited periods of time: behaviour therapy has simply not been in existence long enough to make longer-term studies possible. This is an obvious need, but in view of the great cost of mounting such studies, and the comparative poverty of behaviour therapy as compared with psychoanalysis, such studies are unlikely to be forthcoming in great number in the immediate future.

Much, much more has been done in the way of proof by behaviour therapists in the dozen years or so that behaviour therapy has been officially recognized, than has been done by psychoanalysts and psychotherapists in the seventy years or so of Freudian hegemony. Nevertheless it should be stated quite clearly that much more is required before we can say with any certainty what methods are most appropriate for which patients, under what circumstances, or precisely what the effects are likely to be. Failure to be able to provide all the answers should not be confused with having none of the answers; a good deal is known already, and gives us confidence in the usefulness of behaviour therapy in the treatment of neurotic illnesses.

There are two kinds of study on which this belief rests, and both must be taken in conjunction if we are to arrive at any reasonable estimate of the present position. In the first place we have studies of psychiatric patients, taken from child guidance clinic or mental hospital, and subjected to behaviour therapy; comparison is then made with similar patients treated by psychotherapy or given no treatment at all. Clinical studies of this type are perhaps the most convincing, but they inevitably suffer from certain design difficulties implicit in the manipulation of human beings in trouble; it would be unethical and inhumane to keep a patient in a control group who suddenly got worse, for instance. Similarly, a patient in the experimental group might suddenly show psychotic symptoms, requiring drug treatment; it would be unethical and inhumane not to provide such treatment, even though it might ruin the scientific purity of the research design. We shall be discussing three such clinical studies presently.

An alternative to clinical studies is presented by the so-called experimental or analogue studies, in which we use subjects who are suffering from clearly demarcated single phobias, but who are otherwise not psychiatrically ill and who would normally not have come for treatment. Such phobias and fears as have been studied include snake phobias, spider phobias and fears of public speaking. These can be very strong and disabling, and they are similar to neurotic disorders: nevertheless, they may be sufficiently different from clinical disorders (although I doubt this, and although Freudian theory too would doubt this) to make it dangerous to transfer findings from such neurosis analogues to full-blown neuroses. In actual fact findings from clinical and experimental studies are usually in good agreement, but the danger exists and should be recognized.

Of the three clinical studies to be discussed, the first two were carried out in my own laboratories, while the third has been reported from the University of Southern California. In the first of these, Dr James Humphery carried out a study specifically

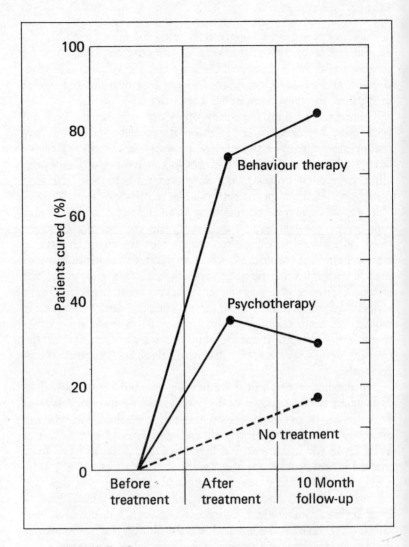

FIGURE 12
Effects of behaviour therapy, psychotherapy and
no treatment on random samples of child patients
at a child guidance clinic.

designed to compare the results of behaviour therapy with those of traditional psychotherapy. Formerly director of a child guidance clinic and a psychotherapist of many years' experience, Humphery was trained in behaviour therapy specifically in order to conduct the investigation. His subjects were 71 children who had been referred to London child guidance clinics for all types of disorders except brain damage and psychosis. The children were divided into matched groups: the 34 in the control group received no treatment of any kind; the 37 children in the treated group were then divided into two groups, one of which received behaviour therapy and the other traditional psychotherapy. A five-point rating scale was used to establish the severity of each child's disorder (his clinical status) and to evaluate the success of the treatment. Each child was rated on this scale at the beginning of the study; the children in the treatment groups were rated immediately after treatment, while those in the control group were rated ten months after the start of the experiment. Experienced psychiatrists, who did not know to which group a child had been assigned, did the rating. The decision to end treatment was made in consultation between Humphery and the psychiatrist assigned to the case. A rise of two or more points on the clinical rating scale was taken as an arbitrary criterion of 'cure'.

All children were again rated ten months later. Of the children who received behaviour therapy, 75 per cent were rated cured at the close of treatment, as compared with only 35 per cent of those who received psychotherapy. At the ten-month follow-up, 85 per cent of those who had received behaviour therapy were rated as cured – an increase of 10 percentage points – but only 29 per cent of those in the psychotherapy group were still considered cured. Of those who had received no treatment at all, 18 per cent were found to be cured.

These results are even more impressive when differences in the length of treatment are taken into account. The children receiving psychotherapy required 21 sessions spread over 31 weeks before it was thought that treatment could be terminated, but those receiving behaviour therapy required only 9 sessions during 18 weeks. Thus behaviour therapy cured twice as many cases as did psychotherapy, and in less than half the number of sessions. By happen-stance, moreover, the children assigned to the behaviour therapy group were the more seriously ill, which would seem to militate against the success of behaviour therapy. On the other hand, since the children given psychotherapy began treatment with a higher clinical-status rating they were less likely to achieve the two-point rise necessary to denote cure. These factors were undoubtedly important in accounting for the startling difference between the two groups. It should be noted, however, that the percentage of cures resulting from psychotherapy in this experiment did not differ from that usually obtained in the clinics involved in the study.

Another study, similar in some ways, was done on adult neurotic patients by Dr P. Gillan. Her patients were outpatients at a mental hospital suffering from serious and complex phobias and anxieties. She formed four groups of eight patients each, matched on relevant variables; these four groups received differential treatment. Those in Group 1 were given desensitization treatment, combining the use of hierarchies with relaxation. Group 2 was given the hierarchies, but no training in relaxation; Group 3 training in relaxation, plus pseudo-therapy (placebo), but no hierarchies. Patients in Group 4 were given dynamic psychotherapy by psychotherapists. (The behavioural treatments were all administered by Dr Gillan herself.) Patients were rated by the therapists involved, by themselves, and also by an independent psychiatrist uncommitted to either approach, and ignorant of the treatment administered to any particular patient. Physiological measures were also taken of the amount of fear produced by the phobic object or objects, or situations, both at the end of therapy and after a follow-up period of three months.

The results of the study were quite clear cut. Desensitization (the combination of the hierarchies with relaxation) was the most successful of all, with hierarchies only, without relaxation, coming second. The placebo treatment (relaxation without hierarchies) and psychotherapy were both significantly inferior. It should be noted that the views of the patients, the independent psychiatrist, and the behaviour therapist coincided closely with respect to degree of improvement; the psychotherapists tended to over-value the effects of their own treatment markedly. This calls in question the usual practice in psychotherapy of allowing each therapist to evaluate his own work. The outcome of this study on adults agrees well with that on children; in both cases we find that behaviour therapy comes out as much more successful than psychotherapy.

In the third clinical study to be mentioned, 94 patients suffering from moderately severe neuroses and personality disorders were accepted for treatment. Patients were assigned either to a waiting list, to a behaviour therapist, or to an analytically oriented psychotherapist. (The control patients were promised therapy in four months' time.) There were three therapists of each persuasion. The results of the study were as follows. At four months, all three groups had improved significantly with respect to the severity of their target symptoms. The treated groups did better than the control group, and although the behaviour therapy group did better than the psychotherapy group, the difference was not statistically significant. On the scale relating to work, the behaviour therapy group did significantly better than either the psychotherapy or no-treatment groups. In respect to social behaviour, only the behaviour therapy and the control group patients improved significantly; psychotherapy patients did not. 'On a rating scale of overall improvement, 93 per cent of the behaviour therapy patients contrasted to 77 per cent of the psychotherapy and wait-list patients were considered either improved or recovered.' At the one-year follow-up, improvement was maintained or continued in most patients. 'The only significant intergroup difference at one year was that the behaviour therapy patients were still significantly more improved on target symptom severity than the control patients.' (In other words, psychotherapy patients were not significantly improved.) There was no evidence of any symptom substitution in any group. 'On the contrary, patients whose target symptoms improved often reported improvement in other, less important symptoms as well.'

Not too much should be made of these three studies. None is free from faults; all are subject to criticisms – indeed, the perfect experiment only exists in the imagination. Nevertheless, all three come to similar conclusions about the effectiveness of behaviour therapy, and the central conclusion is also found in all other studies examined: there is none in which behaviour therapy is inferior to other methods of treatment, such as psychotherapy, or fails to be more efficient than no treatment. Considering the relative youth of behaviour therapy, this is an encouraging out-

come. Much more work is of course needed before certain conclusions can be reached, but the agreement so far reached is most
encouraging – particularly when it is seen from the vantage point
of the experimental studies to be reviewed next.

Experimental studies have several great advantages. Because of
the lesser urgency of the treatment, subjects can be assigned to
different groups with much greater ease. By concentrating on a
single symptom, such as snake phobias, patients become closely
comparable, and can be equated for 'degree of fear'; furthermore,
this can be objectively measured by behavioural or elec-
trophysiological indices. Final outcome can be objectively
measured in the terms of these indices; we can determine how
much more closely the object approaches a snake at the end of
treatment as compared with the beginning, or what effects exposure to a snake has on his autonomic system (as measured by
increased heart-rate, breathing, sweating, etc.)

There have been literally dozens of experiments of this type,
comparing behaviour therapy with various psychotherapeutic
procedures, control and placebo groups, and other types of psychiatric treatments. Only one such study will be mentioned,
namely that reported by Dr Gordon L. Paul from the University
of Illinois. He took the public-speaking situation as his stress condition for arousing anxiety, using for his experiment 96 students
in speech classes at the University, and choosing those out of a
much larger total of 710 students who were most debilitated by
anxiety, and who requested treatment. There were five groups
altogether in the study. Group A was treated by a desensitization
procedure, Group B by means of insight-oriented psychotherapy,
Group C by means of a meaningless placebo method, and Group
D received no treatment at all, although the members were
aware of the existence of the experiment, and filled in questionnaires. Group E, finally, constituted a no-contact group; they
were simply observed, and did not realize that they took part
(after a fashion) in an experiment. (This group was included to
evaluate changes that might be produced by simple awareness of
the existence of an experimental study, and one's participation in
it.)

Five experienced psychotherapists worked individually with
three subjects in each of the three treatment groups for five hours
over a six-week period; post-treatment measures were then ob-

tained on the treated subjects and the no-treatment controls, and follow-up measures on a psychological test battery for all five groups six weeks later. Attitudinal and improvement ratings were obtained from the subjects themselves, and from the therapists. Statistical analyses of the results 'found systematic desensitization consistently superior (100 per cent success); no differences were found between the effects of insight-oriented psychotherapy and the nonspecific effects of the attention-placebo treatment (47 per cent success), although both groups showed greater anxiety reduction than the no-treatment controls (17 per cent). Improvement was maintained at follow-up with no evidence of "symptom substitution".' None of these results were attributable to differences in competence between therapists. It should be noted that these were essentially psychotherapists by training, with a preference for psychotherapy of the analytic type; they had to be specially prepared for the task of administering behaviour therapy procedures, and still retained a preference for psychotherapy, in spite of the outcome of the study! Thus the favourable result of the study cannot be blamed on possible biases on the part of the therapists; in so far as any biases existed, they went in the opposite direction.

The outcome of this study is typical of practically all the other experimental studies in the literature. There is not one which does not show behaviour therapy superior to all forms of psychotherapy, to placebo treatment, or to no treatment at all. There are usually possible criticisms of any particular study, but what is impressive is the unusual agreement between them with respect to their major outcome, and the mutual support they give to (and receive from) the clinical studies mentioned above. All in all, these studies would seem to establish pretty firmly the general conclusion that on the whole behaviour therapy works, and works remarkably well, considering its youth and the very limited opportunities for training which practitioners and experimentalists have had in the past. Much remains to be clarified, and more and better outcome studies are obviously required. Nevertheless, this major conclusion is not likely to be upset by future work.

The critics of behaviour therapy

A number of criticisms and objections have been made in recent years of behaviour therapy and the theories on which it is based, and in all fairness to objectors a brief review of these should be included. Let me begin by stating that quite obviously no scientific theory, and no application of such a theory, can ever be regarded as beyond criticism; even the best-established theories are subject to anomalies, imperfections, and damaging instances of their predictions failing to be confirmed. If this has been found to be so even with the most renowned of theories in physics, such as Newton's theory of gravitation, how much more is it likely to be true of psychological theories, particularly when these are still in their infancy. To expect perfection, or anything approaching it, is unrealistic; consequently criticisms should be eagerly welcomed, as pointing out weaknesses which can be remedied, faults that can be corrected, improvements that can be made in the general structure. It is quite wrong to think that the scientist regards the critic as his enemy; a good critic is the scientist's best friend. It is in this spirit that one ought to look at criticisms, rather than in a spirit of trying to justify the unjustifiable, more appropriate to politicians than to scientists.

Let us take the first criticism, namely that the theories here outlined and the methods based on them, are grossly oversimplified, and do not measure up to the complexity of human nature. This criticism is often extended to cover the basis of behaviour therapy and its supporting theory in animal work. What is said is that rats and even dogs are much too simple organisms to be able to teach us anything about the infinite complexity of human nature. The behaviour therapist is accused of abstracting certain features of conduct from reality, and in so doing losing sight of the totality with which he ought to be dealing. Indeed, it is precisely this habit of attempting to deal in some way with the complexity of the individual, and the totality of his circumstances, which attracts so many people to psychoanalysis; here as in so many other ways psychoanalysis and behaviour therapy are at opposite ends of a continuum. Is this criticism realistic, is it meaningful and does it in any way throw doubt on the value of behaviour therapy?

My own view would be that it does not. There is no doubt that the criticism hits a very real problem, but I believe that it is unjustified nevertheless. Philosophers of science are agreed that what characterizes science above anything else is precisely its tendency to abstraction; the scientist must have the ability to see those aspects of reality which are relevant to his problems, and disregard those which are not. The law of falling bodies takes no note of all sorts of important qualities, such as colour, or shape, or quality; it ruthlessly abstracts just one characteristic (mass) from the complex reality with which it is faced, and formulates laws having regard precisely to this quality and nothing else. This single-mindedness attracts some people, and repels others; it will be remembered how the great German poet Goethe attacked Newton's colour theory, substituting a much more complex and artistic one of his own, precisely because he could not abide the high degree of abstraction in Newton's work. Nevertheless, it was Newton who was right, and Goethe who was wrong. For a scientific theory, the only criterion is whether it works, not whether people find it appealing. To say that a theory works means simply that we can make predictions from it which are borne out by observation and experiment. We do not require from it that it should explain all sorts of events or properties which may appeal to the outsider as important but which are irrelevant to the theory itself.

Thus it is true that man and dog are differentiated from each other in a myriad ways; however this is irrelevant to a theory which states that with respect to a particular characteristic, X, they are sufficiently alike to generalize from the one to the other. However we may object to such a theory on a priori grounds, or because we dislike being compared in this fashion with dogs and rats, nevertheless there is only one way of settling the question; we must make deductions from the hypothesis that dogs and men are alike with respect to X, and then test these deductions. Dogs and men each have an autonomic system, they form conditioned responses, they extinguish these under conditions of response-prevention in the presence of an unreinforced conditioned stimulus. The proof of the pudding, therefore, is in the eating: do we find that humans do in fact extinguish their neurotic symptoms when put in a response-prevention situation? The fact that they do cannot be gainsaid by simply saying that humans are more complicated than dogs; this statement is both true and irrelevant. The only point asserted is that humans and dogs are similar in certain relevant respects, and the evidence bears this out.

A second criticism is often made by what are known as

'cognitive psychologists'; by this is meant that they assert the priority in man of cognitive over other aspects of adjustment. Their point, similar in some ways to that already considered, would be that simple conditioning theory deals with simple stimuli, like bells, buzzers, lights flashing, whereas conditioning in man, if it occurs at all, uses as stimuli meaningful situations and concepts which are far removed from the simple Pavlovian sensations, and require integration through cognitive processes. This may be agreed to at once, and indeed it will be remembered that Pavlov insisted himself on the importance of the second signalling system, which is in essence what these critics refer to as 'cognitive processes'. However, it must be doubtful if recognition of this fact really makes much difference to the theory. For the purpose of exposition it is much easier to refer to simple stimuli, but even in the animal laboratory much work has been done on complex and compound stimuli, and this work can be extended without insuperable difficulty into the human field. This criticism does not call for any profound restructuring of our theory; it merely requires a certain more careful rephrasing of certain aspects of it. This can be done easily in a technical work; in a popular one such as this it does not seem necessary.

Other critics have objected that the results of behaviour therapy are produced, not through the alleged processes of conditioning and extinction, but rather through certain psychoanalytic processes, such as 'transference'. This term is used to suggest that the patient transfers emotions appropriate to certain people, such as his father, to other people, such as the therapist; indeed, it is suggested that 'cure' can only proceed through such transference. What is suggested is that in behaviour therapy, as in psychotherapy, therapist and patient develop a close personal relationship; that this relationship produces a transference, and that this transference is the active ingredient in the treatment. This is an unlikely contingency, for several reasons. In the first place, psychotherapy and psychoanalysis, where one would expect transference to blossom most strongly, have failed to show any beneficial effect on the neurotic; if transference does not produce any success in treatment under these conditions, why should it do so under conditions of behaviour therapy, when opportunities for transference are certainly much restricted?

In the second place, when we compare behaviour therapy with

psychotherapy, as for instance in the Humphery experiment mentioned in the preceding section, it will be noted that he spent twice as much time with each child when doing psychotherapy as when doing behaviour therapy, thus providing much more opportunity for transference to operate. Yet behaviour therapy was successful, psychotherapy was not. This makes it very difficult to see how transference could be the important ingredient that produced the successful outcome in behaviour therapy. The argument simply does not jell.

In the third place, Professor Peter Lang at Wisconsin has shown that behaviour therapy can be carried out by computer, just as well as by a therapist. Using snake phobic subjects, he programmed the computer to administer increasingly anxiety-provoking stimuli, suggest relaxation in the right places, and gradually work its way up the anxiety hierarchy. There was also a panic button on the machine; when the patient found that too much anxiety was being created by the instructions to imagine some anxiety-provoking situation, he simply punched the button, and the computer returned to relaxation and an easier, less anxiety-provoking item. It was found that this method worked just as well as did personal therapy, and it would be difficult to suggest that the patients formed some kind of transference to the computer! I would suggest that this hypothesis is not a very attractive one, and should be disregarded.

In fact, I would suggest that exactly the opposite is true. Whatever success psychotherapy may achieve is likely to be due to the fact that in its methodology it includes certain features of desensitization. Thus the therapist discusses with the patient his hierarchy of problems, often starting with a relatively mild one and working up to the most anxiety-provoking; he may not actively train the patient in relaxation, but tries to be reassuring and in this way promote relaxation; the patient at the end of therapy is required to use his newly-found skills in the outer world, that is, to generalize from therapist's office to his own home and work background. Desensitization is applied amateurishly and without proper intent; nevertheless the elements are there, and may work occasionally, particularly when the therapist is warm, empathic, and reassuring — and we have seen that it is precisely these personality qualities which seem to go with success in psychotherapy.

A more important and relevant criticism is one which I myself have made a number of times, namely that behaviour therapists neglect individual differences between patients in assigning them to different types of behaviour therapy. Professor DiLoreto, of Western Michigan University, has published an interesting and convincing study to illustrate this point. He used three types of behaviour therapy, each applied by two therapists: desensitization, as practised by J. Wolpe, rational-emotional therapy, as practised by Albert Ellis, and client-centred therapy, as practised by C. R. Rogers. Desensitization we have already encountered; it will not be described again here. Rational-emotive treatment teaches that any sustained negative emotion is based on an irrational idea (conditioned?) and without this idea or philosophy the emotion could not endure over time. Thus, its removal and replacement with a more rational idea is the goal of treatment, which consists essentially in challenging these irrational ideas. In client-centred therapy, the therapist attempts to reduce interpersonal anxiety by encouraging the client to experience, in a psychologically safe relationship, the feeling or feelings which have hitherto been too threatening for him to experience freely. It might be argued endlessly whether these two methods are in fact parts of behaviour therapy or not; such a debate would be rather meaningless. Certainly both Ellis and Rogers would maintain that their methods were derived from the rules and laws of general psychology, including learning theory. Provisionally, at least, we may perhaps accept them and demonstrate the importance of personality factors in relation to the outcome of the treatment.

DiLoreto used groups of extraverted and introverted subjects for his study, all the participants being characterized as suffering from high interpersonal anxieties. Subjects were assigned at random to treatments, and certain predictions made with respect to outcome. When the success of the treatment was analysed, it became clear that all three experimental groups did better than various control groups who had not received any treatment. Desensitization did equally well for both extraverts and introverts, and overall therefore surpassed both rational-emotive and client-centred methods of treatment. These two methods, however, differed very significantly with respect to their effect on extraverted and introverted subjects. Extraverts did much better with client-centred therapy, introverts with rational-emotive therapy. Thus personality obviously interacts powerfully with method of treatment. Introverts treated with rational-emotive therapy do as well as those treated with desensitization, as do extraverts treated with client-centred therapy. But introverts treated with client-centred therapy, or extraverts treated with rational-emotive therapy, do as poorly as subjects in the no-treatment controls.

Another example of this very important fact comes from the work of Dr I. Sarason of Seattle. He tried methods of token economy and of modelling with young delinquents, and found that quite different methods were successful with introverted, ineffective, inadequate youths, who responded well to modelling, and with extraverted, sociable, youths, who responded well to token economy treatment. In each case the recidivism rate was reduced by something like 50 per cent over a three-year follow-up period when treatment was appropriate to personality type; when the treatment was inappropriate, however, there was no improvement. This is an important point; we may easily be misled by negative results into thinking that the method used was useless, when really the fault lay in the improper allocation of subjects or patients to treatment not suited to their personalities. Behaviour therapists, like psychotherapists, pay far too little attention to personality differences of this kind; this I think is a legitimate criticism, but of course one which can easily be remedied.

Most serious of all criticisms that have been made of behaviour therapy is perhaps one which alleges that the methods used are not in fact based on laboratory studies and scientific theories, but are rather accidental discoveries without proper academic background. According to these critics, the language of hypothesis and proof is merely camouflage for essentially unrelated and common-sense methods of treatment which have been known for hundreds of years. Many readers may feel that such a criticism is of little interest; if the methods of behaviour therapy work, as they undoubtedly do, then it is relatively unimportant whether or not they derived from scientific theory or from common sense, whether they are grounded in laboratory experiments or in everyday life experiences. To some extent this is a reasonable answer; many medical discoveries of useful treatment preceded any scientific understanding of the diseases in question. As long as it works, why worry about esoteric academic questions? While I have some sympathy with such a reply, I feel that the criticism needs a stronger answer.

Accidental discoveries in medicine are legion, and very useful many of them have proved; nevertheless, the really important discoveries, such as Pasteur's work on microbes and inoculation, while often anticipated in part by chance, nevertheless only assumed their proper status when aligned with a sound scientific foundation in theory and experiment. It is this alignment which provides a focus for further advance, which alone makes the therapy rational and meaningful, and which gives it a background against which to check anomalies and faults. The methods of behaviour therapy would still be useful even if they lacked the scientific background we have outlined in this book; yet their future progress would be much retarded for such a lack, and their status would unquestionably be very much lower. The criticism, if correct, is therefore not one which can be answered quite so cavalierly.

As it happens, however, there is very little in this notion that behaviour therapy grew haphazardly and by a series of lucky accidents. Having myself contributed to its growth, together with colleagues and friends, and knowing most of the active workers in this field personally, I have no doubt that the great majority of them have based their work and much of their inspiration on modern learning theory, on the one hand, and laboratory work with animals and humans on the other. Several examples of this have already been quoted, from the way in which partial reinforcement leads to a reduction in extinction (in the case of the bell-and-blanket method of treatment for enuresis) to the use of escape prevention (in the case of obsessive-compulsive disorders). It is simply not true to say that behaviour therapists have not been influenced by academic theories and by experimental results in their work; such a criticism really tells us that the critic knows little of either the experimental-theoretical or the practical side of behaviour therapy.

There is, however, another way in which this criticism can be understood, and in this sense we might say that it is perfectly justified. The critics might be understood to say that none of our theories are universally accepted; that there is much dispute concerning the interpretation of animal experiments, such as those quoted in this book; that there are many anomalies in our work which defy explanation by current theories; that the steps from theory to application are not as clear-cut and obvious as one might wish; that things do not always work out as one might have thought; and that quite generally the state of perfection has not yet been reached as far as behaviour therapy is concerned. Such criticisms are perfectly justified, and they may lead to a state of humility amply justified in a young science just beginning to establish itself. But these criticisms only prove that we are dealing with an application of scientific knowledge and methodology, not with revealed truths imprinted on stone tablets and brought down to us by ancient prophets. All science is characterized by precisely these difficulties and defaults; no scientific theory is all-embracing, all-powerful, all-true. Even in the hard sciences we find that every theory has to try and explain away anomalies; that there is no universal agreement on important matters; that different explanations are possible of many crucial experiments. We mentioned earlier Newton's theory of gravitation, which used to be looked upon as typical of the perfection of scientific genius; yet from the beginning it was faced with anomalies – Newton could not explain the motion of the moon, and right to the end the precession of the perihelion of Mercury defeated all attempts at explanation in Newtonian terms. Behaviour therapy does not claim to be an exception to this rule; the theories on which it is based are not perfect by any means, and will undoubtedly require refurbishing before we get much nearer to the truth. We have already shown that the universal law of extinction, as found in most textbooks, has to be changed completely in order to accommodate the facts; no doubt there are other equally impressive laws which require change, or which may even have to be abolished. That is the way science works, by conjecture and refutation; there is no absolute certainty, only gradual improvement through criticism, new theories, new deductions. Criticism is valuable when it deals with actual, demonstrable faults in a theory or an experiment, and when it is constructive, suggesting new hypotheses, new experiments, new applications. When it is merely negative, asserting general, non-specific faults of pseudo-philosophical kind, it is not helpful. Unfortunately much of the criticism directed at behaviour therapy has been of that kind.

The ethics of behaviour therapy

There has been much discussion of ethical problems in relation to behaviour therapy, stimulated in the main by two sources. One of these is ideological; it is suggested that psychiatrists and psychologists use these methods merely to shore up and make more tolerable an unjust society. The other is humanitarian – that the methods of behaviour therapy are cruel and inhumane and should not be used. The former criticism is often voiced by the so-called 'anti-psychiatry' psychiatrists like Cooper and Laing; the latter finds expression in such films as 'A Clockwork Orange'. The objections raised on these grounds are largely mistaken; they derive from profound ignorance of the workings of behaviour therapy and the nature of mental illness. Let us take the ideological argument first.

When critics argue that mental disease is a product of a given society, consequent upon a given mode of production, they merely repeat a political slogan which clearly fails to apply to this particular field. Mental disorder, very much like the forms we find in our society, has been recorded in many ancient and primitive societies, and also in communist countries. Clearly these differ profoundly in their modes of production, yet the outcome, as far as mental disorder is concerned, is much the same. How then is it possible for neurotic or psychotic disorders to be due to a specific social organization, based on a specific mode of production (say the capitalist one) when exactly similar disorders are found in countries and ages when capitalism was far from being the social mode? The argument in general terms makes no sense at all, and the prevalence of neurotic and psychotic disorders in the Soviet Union and other communist countries makes it very difficult to accept such notions. Nor is it clear how such a suggestion would work in detail. Just what features of the capitalist system cause a person to develop spider phobias, or obsessive-compulsive symptoms relieved by hand-washing? Was it capitalism that caused Nebuchadnezzar to have a schizophrenic breakdown? It is merely necessary to ask these questions to see that the theory makes no sense at all.

It is possible to see some slight support for it when we turn to sexual disorders, such as homosexuality, and to criminality and other antisocial disorders. Can we justify the treatment of homosexuals, it is asked, when clearly all we are doing is to make their behaviour agree more closely with the ideals of a tyrannical society which has no right to prescribe a person's mode of sexual adjustment? Such an objection, clearly, does not only relate to behaviour therapy, but equally concerns all other types of psychiatric treatment. It is a universal objection, and some 'antipsychiatry' psychiatrists do indeed use it in this broad sense. It would be easy to discuss it in great detail, but like many ethical discussions this one too would probably founder on the difficulty of finding some agreed basis on which such an argument could be conducted. As a famous wit once said when seeing two fishwives shouting at each other across a narrow street from the windows of their living rooms: 'These two will never agree; they are arguing from different premises!'

There is only one argument which I believe to be relevant, and that is the very simple one that *the decision as to the desirability or otherwise of treatment should be left to the patient himself.* Society has no right to force him to undergo treatment, and the therapist has no right to refuse him treatment should he desire it. A number of years ago, a well-known QC approached me after a public lecture I had given in the London Guildhall on the subject matter of behaviour therapy. He asked me if he could be treated for his homosexuality in our department; he had tried psychoanalysis and other methods in vain already. I had to turn him down because we did not at that time have any facilities for such treatment. A few weeks later he hanged himself. If facilities had been available, would I have been justified in turning him down on the grounds that some people's moral ideals suggest that treatment would be unethical? There clearly are problems in cases of this kind, but there are no facile answers. Each case has to be looked at separately, and each decision has to be made by the individual therapist concerned, in agreement with the patient. Obviously it would be wrong to force treatment on an unwilling patient; equally obviously it would be wrong to withhold treatment from a patient eager to be treated. There are intermediate steps on this continuum and it is with them that the problems arise. There can be no general answer.

As far as prisoners are concerned, I would suggest that much the same principle holds. We have already seen that personality is closely concerned with the predisposition to criminality, and that the alleged sociological and ideological causes have a much more doubtful status; criminals in communist countries show much the same personality picture as do criminals in Western countries. Many prisoners would be only too eager to volunteer for a token economy kind of behaviour therapy, were they given the chance. It does not seem particularly ethical to withhold this possibility from them on *a priori*, ideological grounds. Again one could argue this point for a long period of time; I shall leave it to the reader to consider the problem, and furnish his own conclusion. There clearly are two sides to the question, but the notion that most criminals are in some way protesting against an unjust and wicked social system is clearly not true; criminals are if anything more staunchly conservative than their peers outside prison! Crime is not a protest against a social system, and its universal occurrence in all types of social system clearly reveals the emptiness of this dogma.

When we turn to the other ethical argument, which assumes that the methods used are inhumane, we must say at once that the argument is based on factual error. The methods used in 'A Clockwork Orange' are not such as would recommend themselves to any living behaviour therapist, nor are they like anything that has ever been used. The producer has simply misused and misunderstood the principles of aversion therapy in order to sensationalize and make acceptable a picture capitalizing on cruelty and sex; what is shown has nothing to do with behaviour therapy as understood or practised by responsible psychologists. The same is true of much that is written, particularly in the USA, about behaviour modification. Such writers often include drug treatments, or electroshock and leucotomy operations, under this heading, ignorant of the fact that there is simply no connection at all. Readers will remember the accusation that those advocating the bell-and-blanket treatment for enuresis wanted to give electric shocks to the penises of little boys: these more general accusations are as inaccurate and meaningless as that. Of course a film like 'A Clockwork Orange' has a much greater propaganda effect, and reaches far more people, than does the sober truth, written up in scientific journals and books. Nevertheless, such films are nothing but propaganda, inaccurate, oversimplified, and sensationalized; it would not be sensible to pay attention to such worthless material.

Of all the methods of behaviour therapy, it is of course only that of aversion therapy which gives rise to such accusations, and it is important to realize that out of 100 applications of behaviour therapy, less than 1 would involve aversion therapy. Even then, the actual application of physical pain, as in electric shock or apomorphine-induced nausea, is getting more and more rare. Many behaviour therapists now use the method of *covert sensitization*, asking people to associate the image of the activity to be abandoned with a mental picture of something nauseous and disagreeable; this method has been shown to work extremely well, and avoids the use of actual bodily pain. However, I would not like to hide behind this alternative method of treatment; we must face the problem of aversion therapy directly.

Let us take as an example head-bangers. These are children who bang their heads. This sounds a mild and slightly ridiculous kind of conduct, but it is in fact very dangerous and debilitating. Children may lose their sight (the retinas may become detached through the head-banging) and indeed they may kill themselves. What can we do? Orthodox medicine suggests nothing better than simply tying the children up, by roping them to a chair; this is obviously only a palliative, and does not cure them. Furthermore, it cannot be continued for any length of time. Psychoanalysts have suggested that what these children need is more attention and mother love; hence they advise mothers to gather up the child in her arms when he starts to bang his head, and show him plenty of affection. This is more humane, but unfortunately the method rewards the child for doing the thing you do not want him to do – he bangs his head, and immediately afterwards you reward him (give positive reinforcement) for his conduct! One would predict on psychological principles that this method would make things worse, and indeed that is what happens.

The method suggested by psychological theory is exactly the opposite. When the child starts to bang his head, the mother is instructed to pick him up, take him into an empty room, and leave him there for ten minutes, closing the door behind her; this procedure is called 'time out', because during this time the child receives no positive reinforcement of any kind. After ten minutes are up, the mother opens the door again, takes the child back into the living room, without saying anything about the head-banging; the whole affair is forgotten. A few applications of this method of negative reinforcement are usually sufficient to cure the child permanently, without relapses or symptom substitutions. In a few cases something more than 'time out' is required; a mild electric shock may have to be given as added negative reinforcement.

Now the critic might say that we are being cruel to the child; that we punish him for something that is not really his fault, either by withdrawal of love and attention, or even by giving him electric shocks. All very true; but what is the alternative? We can tie him up; or we can smother him with love. The first method does not cure him, and the second makes him worse. Something has to be done; is this mild version of aversion therapy really so terrible? Of course we would prefer some other method that did not involve even the mildest form of 'punishment'; but that is not the alternative at present available. Let the reader put himself, in imagination, into the role of the unfortunate parent, faced with the possible blindness or even death of a loved child; would he not be willing to use the behaviourist's method in preference to the available alternatives? When gangrene has set in, the surgeon will remove the leg to save the patient's life; is this needless cruelty? The dentist drills a cavity in order to insert a filling; do we complain that he is a sadist? We always have the alternative of doing nothing, or doing something ineffectual or counterproductive. But if we have the best interests of the patient at heart, we must do what is best under the circumstances, even if this means inflicting some mild degree of discomfort or pain in order to save him from much greater discomfort or pain. I do not believe that there really exists an ethical or moral problem in the application of behaviour therapy, other than one which is universal in psychiatry and indeed in all medicine.

Readers may not be entirely convinced of this when they recall some of the things done in American prisons in the name of behaviour therapy. The bestial cruelties and assaults upon the dignity of the person perpetrated in some of these prisons were in the tradition of some of the American States which have never taken kindly to the doctrine of humane treatment of prisoners, but they have nothing whatever to do with behaviour therapy nor were any trained behaviour therapists involved. It is unfortunate that newspapers, film makers and other representatives of the media can obfuscate issues by using words and names like behaviour therapy in contexts which have nothing whatsoever to do with the concepts in question, thus confusing beyond hope issues which really are quite simple. The first principle of behaviour therapy is that treatment should not be imposed on the patient, but sought by him on an entirely voluntary basis. It is true that the term 'voluntary' can give rise to difficulties when used in relation to psychotic patients, and that for criminals there may be subtle pressures which may invalidate its use. But as far as the 'Clockwork Orange' type of treatment is concerned, all one can say is that it is so far removed from anything even remotely tolerable in terms of this principle that its contents can have no relation to behaviour therapy, as understood by practitioners and theorists.

In summary, ethical questions are very difficult to deal with because general principles are few and far between. Perhaps Immanuel Kant's categorical imperative may serve as the best guide to behaviour therapists; never treat another human being as a means to an end, but always as an end in himself. The application of this principle may still give rise to problems and difficulties, but then human problems never were easy to solve, or reducible to a formula. Behaviour therapists, in my experience, take a standpoint no less ethical than that characteristic of the medical profession as a whole. They do not necessarily agree on every detail, and in every case; but they are certainly not subject, as a group, to the wholesale condemnation which the creators of such films as 'A Clockwork Orange' have helped upon them.

Postscript: You and Neurosis

This book will have told readers roughly what modern psychology has to say about neurosis, and what modern methods of therapy are like. Those who are themselves suffering from neurotic fears and anxieties, or have some other symptoms of a similar kind, or have relatives or friends who are in a similar predicament (and there are few of us who are not in that position) may ask just how all this relates to their own particular state. Such a question is difficult to answer, but it is put to me so often that I shall attempt to give at least a few hints.

In the first place, we have seen that neurotic disorders are behavioural in nature, not medical. The cure does not consist in tranquillizing pills or other drugs, nor in electroshock or brain surgery of any kind. The former are just palliatives, with serious habit-forming effects and frequent side effects, and the latter are unproven and unjustifiable interference with the physical substratum of the conscious mind. Many sufferers come to the doctor with the implicit attitude: 'Cure me!' This may make sense in the case of physical diseases, but not in the case of neurosis. What can be done by the psychiatrist or psychologist is to create a situation in which, and through which, the patient can cure himself, through developing new habits and extinguishing old ones. Much of the work has to be done by the patient. This is inevitable, and patients who refuse to do the necessary work have to fall back on tranquillizers and other unsatisfactory palliatives. Just as no one can learn French or Latin for you, or practise your tennis or golf shots, so no one can get rid of your hang-ups, your anxieties and phobias, for you. Only you can do that. The teacher, the coach, the psychologist can help you, but he cannot do it for you. This also means, of course, that the patient's cooperation is absolutely vital. You cannot force behaviour therapy on some unwilling victim (even if anyone should wish to do so), simply because without this large element of cooperation the whole thing just would not work.

In the second place, the patient has to make up his mind whether he wishes to be treated along behavioural lines, or by psychotherapy or psychoanalysis. Ideally such a decision should be his entirely, though, as we shall see, there are problems and complications in the way of realizing such a desirable state of affairs. Readers will not be in any doubt as to the recommendation I would make, but many people undoubtedly prefer the 'talking' treatment of the psychotherapist to the 'activity' treatment of the behaviourist, and there is every reason in the world why the choice between the two should be left to the patient. (It would also be advisable, of course, if psychotherapists followed the example of behaviour therapists and told prospective patients quite frankly what they might expect to get out of the treatment – with facts and figures to support their estimates.)

The third point arises if and when the patient opts for behaviour therapy. The simple problem that arises then is that there are very few properly trained behaviour therapists in Britain. There are many more in the USA, but also many more quacks who are trying to cash in on the popularity of behaviour therapy, and call themselves by that name in order to earn a quick buck, in the absence of any proper training. It is unfortunately still true that training courses in psychiatry always include psychotherapy, seldom behaviour therapy, and that even when this is included the background of the psychiatrist typically does not include any proper training in psychology, learning theory, conditioning, etc. We have the absurd situation that men whose main job it will be to treat patients suffering from behavioural disorders by psychological means have to undergo a lengthy training in medical matters, which are totally irrelevant, but receive no, or only the most cursory education in psychology, which is directly relevant! How this situation can be remedied is not for me to say; I merely draw attention to it in order to forewarn readers that their search for a good behaviour therapist will be a lengthy and difficult one, in the absence of any sense of urgency on the part of psychiatry as a whole to train practitioners in this new art.

This leads me to a fourth point, which is that most behaviour therapists are in fact not medically trained psychiatrists, but clinical psychologists lacking a medical degree. Their qualification is a good university degree in psychology, followed by years of training as clinical psychologists in one of the university departments which specialize in this training. Often psychologists practising behaviour therapy work together with psychiatrists and social workers in a psychiatric team, which may be attached to a mental hospital, child guidance clinic, or university department. Such team work is probably the best condition for success, but the number of such teams is pitifully small at the moment. How to locate one will tax any patient's abilities and energy to the utmost. The position is easiest in the USA, much less favourable in the UK, and pretty hopeless in Germany, France, and other European countries. These countries are still under the almost complete sway of psychoanalysts and of Freudian notions, so much so that only the occasional behaviour therapist manages to survive the fierce onslaught on his methods and practice.

It should be noted that what has been said above only applies to neurotic disorders of the type discussed in this book. Psychotic disorders like schizophrenia and manic-depressive illness do require medical expertise and drug treatment, and are properly the field of medically trained psychiatrists. There are many other medical disorders which are usually treated by psychiatrists, although often neurologists are also consulted; these include geriatric disorders, disorders of the brain and the central nervous system, epilepsy, and many others. With these we are not here concerned; although they fill about half of our hospital beds, they are far less numerous than the all-pervasive neurosis. There are not enough psychiatrists to cover these properly medical disorders, leave alone to take on the millions of cases of neurotic disorder. For this reason alone, even if there were not many others, treatment of neurosis should be left to properly trained clinical psychologists, thus leaving the medically trained psychiatrists to look after their own medical responsibilities.

Can a neurotic patient treat himself? In principle the answer should probably be yes, although in practice there are many difficulties. Methods of desensitization and flooding, or even modelling, can be devised by an intelligent person for himself, and with the help of a friend these can be put into practice fairly expeditiously. There is not all that much danger of making things worse; the worst that can happen is usually that there is no improvement. Cases of successful self-treatment have been known, but in my opinion it would usually be very much better to engage the services of a good, experienced behaviour therapist. Unfortunately, as already pointed out, this is not always possible, and if the choice were between self-treatment and psychotherapy I have little doubt which I would choose. However, such a desperate choice should not be necessary, and it is very much to be hoped that in the near future more and more behaviour therapists will be trained so that it can be avoided.

Unless private treatment is desired, and there are now a few behaviour therapists in the private sector, the first step of a prospective patient should be to consult his GP, who will give him a letter to a hospital or consultant. This consultant can then refer him for treatment to a behaviour therapist. If the GP and the consultant do not know at which hospitals behaviour therapy can be administered, the patient might get in touch with the British Association for Behavioural Psychotherapy which has a full list of therapists and their location. The secretary of the British Psychological Society will be in a position to give enquirers the address of the secretary of the BABP at the time of enquiry. The complexity of the procedure is regrettable, but is imposed by the novelty of the procedure and the gargantuan complexity of the Health Service.

It should be stated in this connection that the non-medical nature of the treatment makes it not only possible but advisable for parents, relatives and other persons close to the patient to take part in the treatment, under close supervision by the therapist of course. Clearly desensitization in the hospital environment must be followed or accompanied by desensitization in the home, and the same is true of other methods of treatment. Sexual difficulties of a neurotic nature almost always require the assistance of the spouse or girl-friend; school difficulties the help of the teacher involved. In recent years there has also been a move to use nurses for much of the work involved in behaviour therapy. Once the plan of treatment has been formulated, it can be explained to specially trained nurses and the actual process of desensitization or whatever can be entrusted to them. The evidence to date indicates that this works just as well as treatment by psychologist or psychiatrist, and much increases the interest the nurse takes in his or her work – being able to do something active and obviously curative is a very good incentive and morale booster. In all these way non-academic persons can become involved with the treat-

ment process, and give welcome and often essential help to the
therapist.

Neurosis is a grave affliction, let there be no doubt on that
score. Many patients prefer suicide to continuing life under the
constant threat of anxiety, depression and fear. Yet it is usually
benign, as we have seen, remitting spontaneously after a year or
two in the majority of cases, and in those cases where it does not
remit, treatment is not only possible but will usually be successful
in a fairly short period of time. Unfortunately some treatments,
particularly psychoanalysis, can make the disorder worse, can
bleed the patient of money, energy and hope, and can leave him
addicted to the bought friendship of the analyst. (One recent
writer called psychotherapy the 'prostitution of friendship'; in
other words, instead of telling our troubles to our friends, we pay
the analyst large sums of money to listen to them!) The
neurotic finds himself in a difficult situation, hearing contradictory claims on all sides and being unable to evaluate them.
Furthermore, his disorder makes him desperate for a solution and
yet unable to resist the siren voices of those who solicit his
custom. His critical acumen is fatally weakened by his neurosis.
This makes it all the more important that he should have some insight into his disorder, its causes, its nature and the available
means of treating it. Only this knowledge can enable him to
make the right decision himself.

What can the patient hope to achieve, once he undertakes
treatment which proves successful? Symptomatic treatment, such
as behaviour therapy, will cure him of his major symptoms, and
often also of many minor ones. Therapists usually report that
there is an overall improvement in work, sex and social relations,
over and above the alleviation of the specific symptom or symptoms which are under treatment. But there should be no mis-
understanding: the patient who enters treatment with a particular
kind of personality (say a dysthymic personality) is not going to
emerge a roaring lion of courage or an insensitive rhinoceros. He
will remain a rather sensitive, nervous, introverted person.
Wholesale change of personality is rare and unlikely to occur under any kind of treatment. Indeed, most neurotics do not wish for
such wholesale change; they are reasonably happy with their personality (and may often prefer it to alternative types of personality, such as the brash extravert) provided only that they can get

rid of the particular neurotic fears and anxieties, phobias and compulsions, which make their lives a misery. Psychoanalysis indeed promises to make the patient 'a better person', but leaves it quite unspecified what such a wholesale claim can possibly mean – apart, of course, from furnishing no evidence whatever in favour of its ability to produce such a change. Heredity sets pretty clear limits to any changes we may make and psychologists do not claim to work miracles. Our aims are much narrower than that, but within these narrow, reasonable limits we are now able to extinguish the conditioned emotional responses, and the behavioural activities built on them, which constitute the neurotic symptoms of which patients complain. This is an encouraging beginning for the application of science to human problems.

Bibliography

Bibliography

This list of readings is intended for readers who wish to extend their acquaintance with the matters discussed in the text; it will also in part serve as a set of references for points mentioned there. Books and articles mentioned are given under the chapter heading to which they are relevant; this seemed more convenient than giving them in alphabetical order.

1   The Neurotic Paradox

A book by C. D. Spielberger & I. G. Sarason (Eds), *Stress and Anxiety* (3 Vols, Halsted Press), gives a good overview of the subject; see particularly the chapter by M. Lader on 'The nature of clinical anxiety in modern society'. Any textbook on psychiatry will describe the major syndromes of neurosis, and give case histories illustrating these descriptions. General discussions of the unreliability of psychiatric diagnosis and other topics in the chapter will be found in H. J. Eysenck (Ed.), *Handbook of Abnormal Psychology* (Pitman). The Indian study referred to in the chapter was published by G. M. Carstairs & R. L. Kapur, *The Great Universe of Kota* (Hogarth Press). For a discussion of the different types of neurosis, see H. J. Eysenck, *Case Studies in Behaviour Therapy* (Routledge & Kegan Paul).

2   Causes of Neurosis

For a discussion of demonology, see J. Ehrenwald, *The History of Psychotherapy* (Aronson). The topic of enuresis is well treated by S. H. Lovibond in *Conditioning and Enuresis* (Pergamon Press), while the experiment quoted in the text was reported by W. Finley et al., in *Behaviour Research and Therapy*, 1973, 11, 289-298. On the effectiveness of psychoanalysis and psychotherapy, see H. J. Eysenck, *Handbook of Abnormal Psychology* (Pitman) and S. Rachman, *The Effects of Psychotherapy* (Pergamon Press). On Freud, see H. Ellenberger, *The Discovery of the Unconscious* (Allen Lane), and R. M. Jurjevich, *The Hoax of Freudism* (Dorrance).

The triune brain hypothesis is discussed in detail by P. D. MacLean, *A Triune Concept of the Brain and Behavior* (University of Toronto Press); for more general discussions of biological factors, see J. Gray, *The Psychology of Fear and Stress* (Weidenfeld & Nicolson). See also S. Rachman, *The Meanings of Fear*, for a more popular account (Penguin). Anxiety and conditioning are treated by H. J. Eysenck & S. Rachman, *The Causes and Cures of Neurosis* (Routledge & Kegan Paul) in relation to neurosis specifically. See J. Gray, *Elements of a Two-Process Theory of Learning* (Academic Press) and N. J. Mackintosh, *The Psychology of Animal Learning* (Academic Press) for documentation on the experimental side.

3   A Theory of Neurosis

Many of the early papers mentioned are reprinted and discussed in H. J. Eysenck, *Behaviour Therapy and the Neuroses* (Pergamon Press); see also H. J. Eysenck & S. Rachman, *The Causes and Cures of Neurosis* (Routledge & Kegan Paul). The major reference to the new model of neurosis is in H. J. Eysenck, 'The learning theory model of neurosis – a new approach', published in *Behaviour Research and Therapy*, 1976, 14, 251-268. See also D. J. Woods, 'Paradoxical enhancement of learned anxiety response', published in *Psychological Reports*, 1974, 35, 295-314. For personality and neurosis, see H. J. Eysenck, *The Biological Basis of Personality* (C. C. Thomas) and V. D. Nebylitsyn & J. Gray, *Biological Bases of Individual Behaviour* (Academic Press). For the relationship between conditioning and personality, see H. J. Eysenck (Ed.), *The Measurement of Personality* (Medical and Technical Publishers).

4   Methods of Behaviour Therapy

The classic source here is J. Wolpe, *Psychotherapy by Reciprocal Inhibition* (Stanford University Press). A historical introduction is H. J. Eysenck, *Behaviour Therapy and the Neuroses* (Pergamon). For an extensive and up-to-date account, see E. Bergin & S. L. Garfield, *Handbook of Psychotherapy and Behaviour Change* (John Wiley); this also deals with other methods of behaviour therapy and psychotherapy mentioned. For case histories, see H. J. Eysenck, *Case Studies in Behaviour Therapy* (Routledge & Kegan Paul). Many new case studies and experiments are found in recent issues of the journal, *Behaviour Research and Therapy*, as well as theoretical discussions. For modelling, the best source is A. Bandura, *Principles of Behavior Modification* (Holt, Rinehart & Winston), and the Bergin and Garfield *Handbook* mentioned above. For psychosomatic disorders, see O. W. Hill's *Modern Trends in Psychosomatic Medicine* (Butterworth) and for sexual dysfunctions, see D. & P. Gillan's *Sex Therapy Today* (Open Books).

5 Asocial and Antisocial Behaviour

As an introduction, see H. J. Eysenck, *Crime and Personality*, 3rd. edition (Routledge & Kegan Paul). For the underlying theory, see H. J. Eysenck, *The Biological Basis of Personality* (C. C. Thomas). A good introduction to aversion therapy is given by L. P. Ullmann & L. Krasner, *A Psychological Approach to Abnormal Behavior* (Prentice-Hall); see also H. J. Eysenck, *Experiments in Behaviour Therapy* (Pergamon). Case histories are to be found in H. J. Eysenck, *Case Histories in Behaviour Therapy* (Routledge & Kegan Paul). The classic source for token economies is T. Ayllon & N. Azrin, *The Token Economy* (Appleton-Century-Crofts); brought up-to-date in the Bergin and Garfield *Handbook*. For the Maconochie experiment, see H. J. Eysenck, *Psychology is About People* (Allen Lane); this also describes other applications of the method to criminal behaviour. For a critique, see F. M. Levine & G. Fasnacht, 'Token rewards may lead to token learning', in *American Psychologist*, 1974, 29, 816-820, and replies ibid., 1976, 31, 87-92. For homosexuality, see M. P. Feldman & M. J. MacCulloch, *Homosexual Behaviour* (Pergamon Press).

6 Neurosis and Society

The best account of the effects of therapy is S. Rachman, *The Effects of Psychotherapy* (Pergamon Press); see also H. J. Eysenck (Ed.), *Handbook of Abnormal Psychology* (Pitman). Also referred to in the text are R. Bruce Sloane, et al., *Psychotherapy versus Behavior Therapy* (Harvard University Press), and G. L. Paul, *Insight versus Desensitization* (Stanford University Press). Detailed discussions of criticisms of behaviour therapy are given by H. J. Eysenck in two edited books. One is the Bergin and Garfield *Handbook* already mentioned, the other a book by A. Broadhurst & P. Feldman, *Theoretical and Experimental Bases of the Behaviour Therapies* (J. Wiley). For the role of personality in treatment, see

A. O. DiLoreto, *Comparative Psychotherapy* (Aldine-Atherton). Little of interest has been written on the ethical problem, other than *ex parte* ideological arguments based on little factual information; however, the arguments of the 'anti-psychiatry psychiatrists' are well reviewed by S. Rachman in H. J. Eysenck & G. D. Wilson, *A Textbook of Human Psychology* (Medical and Technical Publishers).

Postscript

Some of the issues here raised are discussed in H. J. Eysenck, *The Future of Psychiatry* (Methuen). Readers who feel I am unduly harsh on psychoanalytic treatment, or who wish to have a first-hand account of what it feels like to be a patient under this type of treatment, may like to read C. York, *If Hopes were Dupes* (Hutchinson). S. Sutherland's book, *Breakdown* (Weidenfeld & Nicolson), should be read by anyone liable to undergo psychiatric treatment; it is written by a leading psychologist, and describes his own experiences in the light of his knowledge of learning theory and the general experimental background of psychiatric treatment.

Index

Index

ability, excluded from consideration of personality, 91
abstraction, as characteristic of science, 188-9
active psychotherapy, 111
adolescence, adolescent behaviour, 105, 142
adoption studies, 145
age, effects of, on personality, 105
Albert B. (case history), 63-5, 72, 77
alcoholism, 151, 153-6, 171
alienation, crime and, 143
analogue studies, *see* experimental studies
analysis, *see* psychoanalysis
animal experiments, relevance of, to humans, 60, 188-9
anti-psychiatry psychiatrists, 173, 196
antisocial behaviour, *see* crime
anxiety, 22-3
  clinical studies of, 184
  desensitization treatment of, 56, 122-3, 180, 184, 187
  drive properties of, 86, 87-8
  in enuretic children, 48
  experimental studies of, 186-7
  free-floating, 122
  lack of appropriate (belle indifference), 22
  lifelong, constitutional, 35
  recovery from, speed of, 171
  see also fear
anxiety state, 22
approach-avoidance conflict, 78-80
Aretaeus the Cappadocian, 38
arousal levels, 104
artists, personality traits of, 98-9
ascending reticular activating system, 104
Ashen, Dr B., 116
asocial behaviour, 150-1
assortative mating, 100-1

asthma, 134
atomic attack, phobia concerning (case history), 116-18
aversion therapy, 152-61, 199
  alcoholism treated by, 153-6
  ancient Greek case of, 152
  cruelty of, alleged, 199-200
  fetishism treated by, 157-9
  head-bangers treated by, 199-200
  homosexuality treated by, 156-7
  mental health and, 155-6
  obesity treated by, 159-60
  punishment contrasted with, 152
  transvestites treated by, 157
Ayllon, Dr Teodoro, 162
Azrin, Dr Nathan, 162

Bandura, Professor Albert, 130-1
Bechterev, V. M., 160-1
bed-wetting, *see* enuresis
behaviour, personality concepts descriptive of, 91-2
behaviour modification (Skinnerian behaviourism), 168-9
behaviour therapists, training and availability of, 203-4, 205
behaviour therapy:
  by computer, 191
  criticisms of, 49-50, 187-95
  effectiveness of, 9, 19-20, 46, 180-7, 190-1, 206-7
  methods of, 107-38; *see also* aversion therapy; desensitization; flooding; modelling
  psychoanalysis contrasted, 47-50, 108-10
  see also Watson, J. B.
bell-and-blanket treatment, 45-50
belle indifference, 22
biofeedback, 135, 136-8

birth dates, pattern of, among psychotics, 18

blanket treatment, of enuresis, *see* bell-and-blanket treatment

Boulougouris, Dr J. C., 127

brain, 51-3, 103-4
  disorders of, 204
  operations on, 104-5, 173

breakdown, nervous, 59

British Association for Behavioural Psychotherapy, 205

British Psychological Society, 205

Burt, Sir Cyril, 142

Bykov, Dr K. M., 137

cancer, lung, 134

capitalism, as cause of crime, 143

cat phobia (case history), 70-2, 81, 82, 83, 113-16

catharsis, *see* flooding

Celsus, 38

Chave, Dr J., 31

chemical malfunctioning:
  neurosis not due to, 17
  psychosis and, 17, 18

Cheyne, G., 27

children:
  antisocial behaviour in, 141, 142
  clinical studies of, 183-4
  upbringing of, 167

choice, neurotics and, 24-5

Cicero, Marcus Tullius, 42-3

cleaning, *see* washing

client-centred therapy, 192-3

climate, as cause of neurosis, 27

clinical studies, clinical trials, 41-2, 170-5, 181, 181-6

'Clockwork Orange, A', 196, 198, 201

cognition, *see* thought

cognitive psychologists, 190

colitis, ulcerative, 134

communist countries:
  crime in, 143-4, 198
  neurosis in, 196

communists, paranoia concerning (case history), 169

complexes, 12, 38-9, 41, 107-8

compulsive behaviour, *see* obsessive-compulsive behaviour

computer, behaviour therapy by, 191

conditioned response, 108
  conscience as, 146-7
  criminals' failure to form, 151, 152
  drive properties in, 85-8
  extinction of, 47-9, 58, 81-2, 83-5, 87-8
  incubation of, 83-5, 87-8, 123-4
  strength of, in neurosis, 82-3
  see also conditioning

conditioned stimulus (CS), 43, 45-6, 55-8 *passim*, 87, 123
  choice of, preparedness and, 77

conditioning, 45, 53-5, 58-9
  Albert B. (case history), 63-5
  cat phobia (case history), 70-2, 81, 82, 83, 113-16
  cognitive processes and, 190
  of extraverts and introverts, 146-7
  impotence (case history), 69-70
  parameters of, 76-7, 152-3
  preparedness and, 76-8
  traumatic, 76, 78, 82
  two kinds of, 160-1; *see also* instrumental conditioning
  Watson's theory of, 74-6

conflict, 78-80
  approach-avoidance, 78-80
  aversive effects of, 78
  nervous breakdown induced by, 59

conscience, 146-7

contamination, fear of, *see* washing

continuous reinforcement, *see* reinforcement, continuous or intermittent

contract, in token economy, 163

control groups, controlled experiments, 41-2, 171-3, 175

conversion symptoms, 22

Cooper, Dr D. G., 196

coronary disease, 134

counter-conditioning, 112; *see also* desensitization

Cox, Dr D., 135

crime, criminality, 106, 140
  causes of, 143-9

criminals:
  adolescent, 105, 142

conditioned responses lacking in, 151, 152
personality traits of, 98, 106, 140-2
treatment of, 196, 197-8; *see also* prison
Crisp, Dr A. H., 159
cruelty, behaviour therapy accused of, 196, 198-201
CS, *see* conditioned stimulus
cure:
  alcoholism, 153-6
  enuresis, 46
  homosexuality, 156-7
  patient's role in, 202
  see also behaviour therapy, effectiveness of; clinical studies; psychoanalysis, effectiveness of; psychotherapy, effectiveness of; remission, spontaneous; treatment

Dalton, John, 62
decadence, as cause of neurosis, 27
delinquents, young, 193; *see also* adolescence
Demosthenes, 152
depression, 15, 19
desensitization, 56, 65, 66, 69, 110-23, 192
  anxiety treated by, 56, 122-3, 180, 184, 187
  phobic fears treated by, 67-8, 113-21, 180, 184
  psychotherapy may include, 191
  sexual problems treated by, 121-2, 157
diabetes mellitus, 134
diagnosis, diagnostic methods, variations in, 20-1
diathesis, diathesis-stress continuum, 35, 89
DeLoreto, Professor A. O., 192
dirt, fear of, *see* washing
disease:
  causes of, 38
  neurosis as, 34-5
doctors, general practitioners, neurotic patients and, 29-30, 31-2, 34-5
dogs:
  conditioning of, 45, 58-9, 149; *see also* shuttle-box experiment
  humans differentiated from, 189

training of, 166
dominance, directional, 90
dream interpretation, 39, 41, 109-10
drive (motivation), 56
  conditioned response and, 85-8
  neuroticism and, 149
drug taking, 151
drug treatment, 34, 104, 204
dummy treatment, *see* placebo treatment
dysthymia, 22, 106, 140, 151, 152

E, *see* extraversion-introversion
electroshock treatment (ECT), 173
Ellis, Dr Albert, 192
endogenous depression, 19
English Malady, The (Cheyne), 27
enhancement, of conditioned response, *see* incubation
enuresis (bed-wetting), 40-50
environment:
  neurotic behaviour influenced by, 19, 31-2
  personality influenced by, 99, 105
  pyschotic behaviour rarely influenced by, 19
  Watson's view of, 65
epilepsy, 204
Erbkreise (genetic circles), 18
erection, sexual, 70
Essen-Möller, Dr E., 30
ethical problems, in treatment, 151, 173-4, 196-201
evoked potentials, 18
evolution, 51-3, 75
exorcism, 37, 38
experimental studies (analogue studies), 181, 186-7
expressive tests, 102
extinction, of conditioned responses, 47-9, 58, 81-2
  in alcoholism, 154
  incubation and, 83-5, 87-8, 123-4
extraversion, 21-2, 95, 104-6
extraversion-introversion (E; personality dimension), 94-5; *see also* introversion
extraverts, 140
  conditioning of, 146-7
  criminals tend to be, 106, 142-9

psychotherapy and, 179
types of therapy suited to, 192-3

fear, 22-3, 74-7
  build-up of, in neurosis, 82-3, 88
  drive properties of, 86, 87-8
  innate, 74-7
  see also anxiety; phobias
fetishism, 86, 151, 157-9
flooding (response prevention, catharsis,
    implosion), 57, 69, 123-30
  duration of exposure to, 123-4
  obsessive-compulsive behaviour treated
    by, 124-30, 180
  Watson's view of, 65, 66
free-floating anxiety, 122
Freeman, Dr H. L.,70, 113
Freud, Sigmund, 14, 17, 38-40, 107, 109,
    138; *see also* psychoanalysis
Freundlich, Dr A., 135
frustrative non-reward, 78, 80
functional psychosis, *see* psychosis

Galen, 92
Gallup Poll Organization, 32
general practice, practitioners, *see* doctors
genetic circles (Erbkreise), 18
genetic predisposition, *see* heredity
genotype, 102
geriatric disorders, 204
Gillan, Drs P. and R., 121, 184
glass, broken, phobia concerning (case
    history), 118-21
Goethe, Johann Wolfgang von, 189
graphology, 102

habit deficiency, 43-4; *see also* con-
    ditioning
Hagnell,·Dr A., 30
handbags (fetishism case history), 158-9
Haslam, Dr M. T., 118
headaches (case history), 135-6
head-bangers, 199-200
Heinroth, Dr E., 138
'hello-goodbye' effect, 177
heredity, genetic predisposition:
  neurosis due to, 31, 35

personality influenced by, 99-102,
    105-6
Herzberg, Alexander, 111
hierarchies, of anxiety stimuli, 113,
    117-18, 184
Hippocrates, 92
Hodgson, Dr R., 124, 131
homosexuality, 150-1, 156-7, 171, 196-7
humours, ancient theory of, 92
Humphery, Dr James, 181-3, 191
Huxley, T. H., 10
hypertension, 134
hysteria, hysterical personality, 21-2, 106,
    140

imitation (behaviourist technique), *see*
    modelling
implosion, *see* flooding
impotence (case history), 69-70
incubation (enhancement), of con-
    ditioned response, 83-5, 87-8, 123-4
India, neurosis in, 33
individual differences, role of, in origins
    of neurotic behaviour, 65, 72, 78,
    88-9, 105-6
inferiority, constitutional, 65, 89-90
inhibition, reciprocal, 112; *see also* desen-
    sitization
innate fears, 74-7
insight:
  neurotics characterized by, 16
  psychotics' lack of, 17, 21
Institute of Psychiatry (London Univer-
    sity), 111
instrumental (operant) conditioning,
    160-1, 168-9
intelligence, 90, 91
intermittent reinforcement, *see* reinforce-
    ment, continuous or intermittent
introversion, 21, 22-3, 94-5, 104-6
introverts:
  conditioning of, 146-7
  psychotherapy and, 179-80
  types of therapy suited to, 192-3

Janet, Pierre, 21
Jaspers, Professor, K., 37
Jenner, Edward, 38

job selection, personality and, 98-9
Jones, Professor H. Gwynne, 137
Jones, Mary Cover, 66-9
Jung, Carl Gustav, 14, 21, 22, 94, 98, 140

Kant, Immanuel, 201
Kendrick, Dr D. C., 70, 113
Kota, 33

Lader, Dr M., 33-4, 35
Laing, Dr R. D., 196
Lang, Professor Peter, 191
learning theory, 11, 47-9
leucotomy, 104-5, 173
Lewin, Dr K., 78
limbic system, limbic lobe, 52-3, 103-4
lobotomy, 104-5

MacLean, Dr Paul, 51-2
Maconochie, Alexander, 164-6
manic-depressive psychosis, 17, 204
marriage, 100-1, 167
Masserman, J. H., 59-60, 111-12
Masters and Johnson, sex therapy of, 122
Maudsley Hospital, 111, 116
Medawar, Sir Peter, 13
medical treatment, 34-5, 203-4; *see also* doctors
menstrual disturbances, 134
mental health, aversion therapy and, 155-6
mental hospitals, neurosis in, 28
metabolic system, *see* chemical malfunctioning
Meyer, Dr R., 135
Meyer, Dr V., 159
migraine, 134
Miller, Dr N., 78
modelling, 66, 69, 130-4
  case histories of, 67-8, 121, 125-6, 131-2
  introverts treated with, 193
Morbid Anxiety Inventory (MAI), 32
motivation, *see* drive
Murphy, Dr H. B. M., 179-80

N, *see* neuroticism
Napalkov, Dr S. V., 84, 88

National Health Service, 34; *see also* doctors
negative reinforcement, *see* reinforcement, positive and negative
nervous system, in neurotics and psychotics, 18
neural reactivity, 18
neurosis:
  causes of, 37-60 *passim*, 87, 108; *see also* conditioning, conflict, etc., *below*
  conditioning, as origin of, 65-6, 108
  conflict, as origin of, 78-80
  fear of, 24
  heredity, genetic predisposition, and, 31, 35
  historical occurrence of, 26, 27
  individual differences, role of, in causing, 65, 72, 78, 88-9, 105-6
  meaning of, 15
  in mental hospitals, 28
  metabolic system not responsible for, 17
  neuroticism and, 105-6
  in non-Western cultures, 33
  normality-neurosis continuum, 16, 26
  pain reactions, as origin of, 78
  prevalence of, 9, 25-35
  psychosis distinguished from, 16-20
  Skinnerian behaviourism and, 168, 169
  stress, as cause of, 9, 25-7, 35, 89
  trauma, as cause of, 76, 78, 82
  treatment of, *see* treatment
  varieties of, 15-16, 20-4
  wartime, 28-9, 35, 76, 78
neuroticism (N), 89-90, 94, 104, 105-6
  criminals and, 142, 149-50
neurotics:
  choices, perverse, of, 24-5
  doctors consulted by, 29-30, 31-2, 34-5
  environment, influence of, on behaviour of, 19, 31-2
  exaggerated emotions characteristic of, 23
  insight characteristic of, 16
  paradoxical behaviour of, 24-5, 53
  personality traits of, 98, 141
  priests etc. consulted by, 34-5, 37, 170-1
  reality testing by, 57-8

treatment of, *see* treatment
non-Western cultures, neurosis in, 33
Norfold Island, 164-6
normality, neurosis and, 16
Nye, Dr J., 44-5

obesity (case history), 159-60
obsessive-compulsive behaviour, 15, 23,
  56, 171, 180
  case histories of, 124-30, 131-2
Oedipus complex, 38, 107
operant conditioning, *see* instrumental
  conditioning
overcrowding, as cause of neurosis, 27
overlearning, 48-9

pain responses, as origin of neuroses, 78
paradox, the neurotic, 24-5, 53
paranoia, 21, 169
parasympathetic system, 70, 103-4
parents, disguised hostility to, 40-1
Pasteur, Louis, 14
patient, treatment of:
  depends on his cooperation, 202
  role of relatives etc. in, 205
  self-treatment, 204-5
  to be voluntary, 197, 201, 203
Paul, Dr Gordon L., 186
Pavlov, Ivan Petrovich, 45, 53, 54, 58,
  58-9, 76, 160, 190
penis plethysmograph, 86
perambulators (fetishism case history),
  158-9
persecution fears, *see* paranoia
personality:
  ancient Greek view of, 92
  brain structure and, 103-4
  four temperaments, modern theory of,
    92-9
  heredity and, 99-102, 105-6
  individual differences, neurosis and, 65,
    72, 78, 88-9, 105-6
  psychologists' use of the term, 90-2
  questionnaires, 95-8
personality disorders, 106, 140, 141, 171,
  185
phenotype, 102

phobias, phobic fears, 15, 22, 76-7, 171,
  180
  atomic attack (case history), 116-18
  broken glass (case history), 118-21
  cats (case history), 70-2, 81, 82, 83,
    113-16
  clinical studies of, 184-5
  evolution and, 75
  experimental studies of, 181, 186
  groups of, 72-4
  growth of, over time, 82-3, 88
  neurosis stemming from, 76
  preparedness and, 76-7
  snakes, 130-1, 186, 191
  Watson's theory of, 65-6
placebo treatment, 41-2, 45, 174, 175,
  184, 187
Planck, Max, 12-13
Plato, 39
Plutarch, 139, 152
positive reinforcement, *see* reinforcement,
  positive and negative
possession, demonic, 37
poverty, crime and, 143
preparedness, 76-8
priests etc., neurotics' recourse to, 34-5,
  37, 170-1
prison, 142
  Norfold Island, 164-6
projective tests, 102
psychasthenia, 22, 140; *see also* dysthymia
psychoanalysis, 13, 38-40
  behaviour therapy contrasted, 47-50,
    108-10
  duration of, 177
  effectiveness of, 42, 107-8, 176-9, 183
  enuresis treated by, 40-1, 42, 47-8
psychopaths:
  adoption studies of, 145
  birth date pattern among, 18
  conditioned responses lacking in, 151,
    152
  criminals and, 140-1
  extraversion and, 22
  spontaneous remission rare among, 171
psychopathy (sociopathy), 106, 140-1
psychosis, 16-17
  chemical malfunctioning and, 17, 18

neurosis distinguished from, 16-20
prevalence of, 17, 30
see also psychotics; schizophrenia
psychosomatic symptoms/disorders, 22,
    134-9
psychotherapy, 12
    active, 111
    behaviour therapy contrasted, 108-10
    clinical trials lacking in, 175-6
    desensitization in, 191
    duration of, 177
    effectiveness of, 10, 19-20, 42, 107-8,
        176-80, 183-7, 190-1, 206
psychotics:
    birth date pattern among, 18
    environment does not alter behaviour
        of, 19
    genetic groups of, 17-18
    insight lacked by, 17, 21
    neural reactivity of, 18
    treatment for, 19, 204
    see also psychosis
public speaking, 186-7
punishment:
    conditioning contrasted, 152-3
    reward and, *see* reinforcement, positive
        and negative
    variable consequences of, 162

questionnaires, personality, 95-8

Rachman, Dr S., 86, 124, 131, 176
rational-emotive therapy, 192-3
Raymond, Dr M. J., 157
Rayner, Rosalie, 61; *see also* Watson, J. B.
reactive depression, 19
reality testing, 57-8
reciprocal inhibition, 112; *see also* desen-
    sitization
regression, Freudian theory of, 17-20
reinforcement, continuous or intermit-
    tent, 46-7, 49; *see also* conditioned
    stimulus
reinforcement, positive and negative, 24,
    162-7
relaxation, in behaviour therapy, 113, 184
remission, spontaneous, 41, 81, 134, 170-3
repression, 109

response, conditioned, *see* conditioned
    response
response prevention, *see* flooding
reward:
    frustrated, 78
    punishment and, *see* reinforcement,
        positive and negative
rheumatoid arthritis, 134
Rogers, Dr C. R., 192
Rorschach test, 102

Sarason, Dr I., 193
schizophrenia, schizophrenics, 17, 20-1,
    166, 204
science, scientific theories:
    abstraction characteristic of, 188-9
    'rightness' of, 47, 62, 188, 194-5
    supersession of old by new, 12-13
    systematic study the basis of, 11, 109,
        193-5
second signalling system, 53-4, 190
sedation threshold, 18
Seligman, Dr M., 76
sensitization, covert, 199
sex, drive properties of, 86-7
sexual aberrations, 151, 196-7; *see also*
    fetishism; homosexuality; transvestites
sexual problems:
    biofeedback and, 136
    desensitization used in treatment of,
        121-2, 157
    erection process, 70
    impotence (case history), 69-70
    psychosomatic illness and (case
        history), 138
Shepherd, Dr M., 29
shuttle-box experiment, 54-8, 87, 123
Skinner, Professor B. F., Skinnerian
    behaviourism, 161, 162, 168-9
Smith, Rev. Sidney, 164
snake phobia, 130-1, 186, 191
society, social pressures:
    crime and, 143, 198
    neurosis and, 25-7, 196
sociopathy, *see* psychopathy
Solomon, Professor Richard L., 147-9
stimulus, *see* conditioned stimulus; un-
    conditioned stimulus

stimulus generalization, 59, 64, 66
stimulus and response, faulty connection
    between, 44; *see also* conditioning
stress, as cause of neurosis, 9, 25-7, 35, 89
suggestibility, as a factor in treatment, 37,
    41-2, 45, 174
Sweetser, William, 138
sympathetic system, 70, 103-4
symptom substitution, 48, 110
symptoms:
    Freudian and behaviourist theories of,
        12, 38, 107-8, 109
    physical, of mental origin, *see* psy-
        chosomatic symptoms
syphilis, fear of, 127, 128

TAT test, 102
Taylor, Dr W., 31
temperaments, theory of the four, 92-9
tests:
    projective and expressive, 102
    psychological, neurotics and psychotics
        distinguished by, 19-20
theories, scientific, *see* science
thought, cognitive (second signalling
    system), 53-4, 190
token economy, 161-7, 193
tonsillectomy, 173 *note*
training, faulty, 43-4; *see also* con-
    ditioning
transference, 110, 190-1
transvestites, 157
traumatic conditioning, 76, 78, 82
treatment, 202-7

cause of disorder and, 37-8
    medical, 34-5, 203-4
    suggestibility and, 37, 41-2, 45, 174
    to be voluntary, 197, 201, 203
    see also behaviour therapy, effectiveness
        of; clinical trials; conditioning;
        cure; doctors; psychoanalysis,
        effectiveness of; psychotherapy,
        effectiveness of
tuberculosis, pulmonary, 134
twins, 99-102, 144-5

ulcer, peptic, 134
unconditioned stimulus (US), 43, 45
unconscious, the, 38-40, 139
urination, frequent (case history), 137-8
urticaria, 134
US, *see* unconditioned stimulus

visceral brain, *see* limbic system

wallpaper, as conditioned stimulus (case
    history), 70
wartime neurosis, 28-9, 35, 76, 78
washing (cleaning, contamination),
    obsession with, 15, 23, 56 case
    histories of, 124-30, 131-2
Watson, J. B., 61-6, 69, 72, 74, 78, 81
weakness, emotional excess as cause of,
    22; *see also* dysthymia
Wolpe, Dr Joseph, 110-13, 192
women, neurosis among, 28, 29, 30, 31,
    32, 33
Wundt, W., 93